Hospital Transports

A Memoir of the
Embarkation of the Sick and Wounded
from the Peninsula of Virginia in the Summer of 1862

Edited and with an Introduction by

Laura L. Behling

State University of New York Press

Published by
State University of New York Press, Albany

Printed in the United States of America

For information, address the State University of New York Press,
90 State Street, Suite 700, Albany, NY 12207

Production by Marilyn P. Semerad
Marketing by Susan M. Petrie

Library of Congress Cataloging-in-Publication Data

Hospital transports : a memoir of the embarkation of the sick and wounded from the peninsula of Virginia in the summer of 1862 / edited by Laura L. Behling.

p. cm.

Originally published: Boston : Ticknor and Fields, 1863.

Letters and papers compiled by Frederick Law Olmsted at the request of the United States Sanitary Commission.

Includes bibliographical references and index.

ISBN 0-7914-6369-9 (alk. paper)—ISBN 0-7914-6370-2 (pbk. : alk. paper)

1. United States Sanitary Commission. 2. United States—History—Civil War, 1861–1865—Hospitals. 3. Hospital ships—United States—History—19th century. 4. Hospital ships—Virginia—History—19th century. 5. Transports—United States—History—19th century. 6. Transports—Virginia—History—19th century. 7. United States—History—Civil War, 1861–1865—Medical care. 8. United States—History—Civil War, 1861–1865—Personal narratives. 9. Medical personnel—United States—Correspondence. 10. Peninsular Campaign, 1862. I. Olmsted, Frederick Law, 1822–1903. II. Behling, Laura L., 1967–

E631.Z5H67 2005
973.7'76—dc22 2004048167

10 9 8 7 6 5 4 3 2 1

Hospital Transports

Contents

Acknowledgments

The tensions that ultimately would lead to the American Civil War were beginning to rumble throughout the North and the South when the Ladies Library Association of Kalamazoo, Michigan, was organized in 1852. Established with the purpose of maintaining a circulating library in order to promote cultured learning, the association contracted to build the still-standing Queen Anne–style edifice for $8,000. The lending library opened its doors November 27, 1878, at 333 South Park Street, and there it stands today. In the more than one hundred and fifty years since its founding, the association has amassed a remarkable and eclectic collection of fiction and nonfiction, collections of poetry, histories, travelogues, and an 1863 copy of *Hospital Transports,* from which this text is reprinted. I am indebted to the Ladies Library Association, not only for graciously allowing me to work with the book, but for providing an elegant repository for the collection, and most importantly, for recognizing the cultural value of the written word.

Thanks also to the Library of Congress Geography and Map Division, Washington, D.C., and the Perry Casteñada Library Map Collection at the University of Texas at Austin for maintaining important collections of historical maps and allowing me permission to include some here, and to the reviewers' careful comments. Most of all, though, the volunteers on the hospital transports ships in 1862 deserve appreciation, not only for enduring a grueling summer on the humid Virginia Peninsula as they tended to the sick and injured, but for their insistence on writing letters home so that the Ladies Library Association could add the original manuscript to its shelves, and so that today we can return to their words in order to better glimpse the horrors and healing of war.

Part One

Editor's Introduction

"making the best of a bad case"

The American Civil War's Battle of Fair Oaks/Seven Pines at the end of May in 1862 almost proved to be more than the United States Sanitary Commission's (USSC) volunteer medical corps could handle. On May 31, Joseph E. Johnston's Confederate army attacked part of General James McClellan's forces north of the Chickahominy River near Fair Oaks/Seven Pines.[1] The Union army's casualties poured into White House in the ensuing days, and like other situations in which the USSC found itself on the Virginia peninsula during the humid summer of 1862, the scene after the battle was chaotic and disorganized as horrendously wounded soldiers were strewn everywhere. The U.S. Army's Medical Bureau brought in its hospital transport ships,[2] but no one was appointed to take charge of them, no one to receive the wounded at the station, no one to transport them properly to hospitals in Washington or Boston, and no one to ensure that the boats had proper stores of medical supplies, food, and water. The commission performed its work as best it could, not from any mandate, but simply by the "right of charity." "Night and day its members worked," one of the nurses reports, "not, you must remember, in its own well-organized service, but in the hard duty of making the best of a bad case."

The confusion about the lack of supplies, however, paled in comparison to the atrocities of the physical conditions of the sick and wounded and the lack of adequate organization on the part of the Medical Bureau to care for the wounded. USSC personnel were confronted with "Men in every condition of horror," a nurse details, "shattered and shrieking, [they] were being brought in on stretchers, borne by contrabands, who dumped them anywhere, banged the stretchers against pillars and posts, and walked over the men without compassion." The men had "mostly been without food since Saturday," she adds, "but there was nothing on board for them," and the cook, to add one final insult to the injuries, "was only engaged to cook for the ship, and not for the hospital." With resources stretched thin, the USSC personnel turned to what they knew best: a philosophy of benevolent care best practiced through order and efficiency.

Despite the horrors of shattered bodies around them, the men and women on the Sanitary Commission's hospital transport ships immediately began ministering to the soldiers' needs. "The first thing *wounded* men want is lemonade and ice," one nurse carefully notes, whereas she adds parenthetically that "with the sick, stimulants are the first thing." Once all the men have had something to drink, then they receive tea and bread. The key, the benevolent woman writes, "was to keep calm ourselves, and make sure that each man . . . was properly refreshed and fed." Throughout the night of June 5, hospital transport ships worked in torrential rain to remove the wounded from the shore. "We went to bed at daylight with *breakfast* on our minds," she concludes, but adds "At half past six we were all on board the *Webster No .2*,[3] and the breakfast of six hundred men was got through with before our own." Despite these desperate conditions, the USSC was able to triage and transport on their ships between two and three thousand men, nine-tenths of whom were fed and cared for exclusively by the Sanitary Commission.

The Battle of Fair Oaks/Seven Pines stretched the human resources and material supplies of the United States Sanitary Commission to its breaking point, but the USSC volunteers responded to the horrors with a meticulous discipline of care, as they had done in the weeks leading up to this battle. "I am not afraid to say," boasted a volunteer nurse during the Civil War, "that no enterprise ever deserved better of the country than this undertaken by the Sanitary Commission. Alive to the true state of things, ever aiming at the best thing to be done, and striving to bring everything to bear upon that, it has already fulfilled a great work." The pride in the "great work" of the United States Sanitary Commission, a civilian organization staffed by administrators from the private sector and volunteer nurses, was to assist the U.S. Army's medical corps in the care and treatment of Union soldiers. The commission evolved from the Women's Central Association of Relief of New York (WCAR), a large grassroots organization devoted to assisting the Union army by collecting supplies, food, and monetary donations. The WCAR approached Henry W. Bellows, a Unitarian minister who was keenly interested in social reform, and Frederick Law Olmsted, who had made his name in public works, to become spokesmen for the association so that it could develop a more pronounced and visible role in the Union's war effort. In a letter to the war department on May 18, 1861, Bellows writes that the conflict that divided the North from the South was "essentially a people's war." Men were volunteering to fight, women were offering their domestic abilities to the cause. "Ought not this noble and generous enthusiasm be encouraged and utilized" Bellows asked, by allowing these volunteer associations to assist the Medical Bureau of the U.S. government? (Sanitary Commission No. 1 1–2)

Less than one month later, President Abraham Lincoln signed the order creating the United States Sanitary Commission, what he called the "fifth wheel" of the U.S. Army's "wagon" (Censer 5). The "wagon" of the army at this time, according to William Quentin Maxwell, was "limping along on three wheels"—the quartermaster's services, the commissary, and the transportation services—while the fourth, the medical and surgical wheel, was only the "little, rickety, antiquated, [and] incompetently led" Army Medical Bureau (Maxwell vi) that was unable to solve the problems of sanitation and hygiene in the Union army. Enlisted men traveled in cattle cars that lacked even the most basic accommodations for human comfort. Food rations often were not healthy, even rancid. Thin blankets did little more than cover beds of rotting straw. The disease rate was rising due to these unhealthful living and traveling conditions, but "the government was helpless to provide adequate precautions" (Maxwell 5). Teenage regimental musicians, cooks, and other noncombatants often served as stretcher bearers and, as James McPherson notes, "More often than not these men and boys bolted in panic when the fighting became hot." The wounded would remain on the battlefields for days at times without medical care, food, or water (McPherson 418). The Northern army during the Civil War, Lori D. Ginzberg succinctly notes, was infamous for its "notorious inefficiency" (154).

Enter the volunteers of the Unites States Sanitary Commission, who advocated for an organized ambulance corps as well as other reforms. The mission of the USSC, the only civilian organization to receive official government sanction (Giesberg vii), was to aid the Union forces until the army's small, antiquated Medical Bureau could better do so on its own (Censer 1). The USSC proposed only "to strengthen the present organization" of the Medical Bureau and was "not intended to interfere with [it]" (*Works and Purposes* 4). They sought to examine, modify, and improve the army's health and fitness by focusing on "Diet, Cooking, Cooks, Clothing, Tents, Camping Grounds, Transports, [and] Transitory Depots." In short, according to the USSC's own history, it would oversee "everything appertaining to outfit, cleanliness, precautions against damp, cold, heat, malaria, infection; crude, unvaried, or ill-cooked food, and an irregular or careless regimental commissariat" (*Sanitary Com-*

mission 6). To carry this out, the U.S. Sanitary Commission recruited surgeons, enlisted men and women as volunteer nurses, and employed the help of "contraband," escaped slaves, under the rallying cry of fulfilling their civic duty.[4] "Although the Civil War did not produce any striking advances in medical knowledge," McPherson argues, "it did generate important innovations in army medical care. Inadequate and amateurish in 1861, the medical services greatly expanded and professionalized by 1863" (418). The USSC, to their credit, engineered and exemplified many of these improvements, and modeled orderliness, cleanliness, and methodical tracking of supplies and personnel for the hapless U.S. government's medical corps.

Just as remarkable as the improvements in hygiene and health was the way in which the USSC accomplished these improvements. The commission was able to organize seven thousand soldiers' aid societies in towns and villages throughout the North and West to support its work during the Civil War. Twelve major regional branches administered this network of local organizations, and although the national administrators were overwhelmingly men, Judith Ann Giesberg explains that the "branches were run by women with a variety of backgrounds and skills" (5). The Sanitary Commission was, in short, a vast network of good-hearted civilians, donating time, money, supplies, and energy—all of which were remarkably ordered through the national organization headquartered in Washington D.C. It was both a grassroots campaign and a national web, efficiently run, altruistically motivated, and guided by one principle as articulated in *Hospital Transports*: "that every man had a good place to sleep in, and something hot to eat daily, and that the sickest had every essential that could have been given them in their own homes."

"Atlantic floating hospitals"

No where was this promise of the USSC made more difficult to ensure than when the war shifted from the banks of the Potomac River to the Virginia Peninsula, when General George B. McClellan launched his offensive against the Confederate capital, Richmond, Virginia, in the spring of 1862. The Confederate army had evacuated Yorktown on May 4; Williamsburg fell to the Union army on May 5, and on May 15, McClellan set up headquarters on the Pamunkey River. Eventually, McClellan's Army of the Potomac pushed slowly up the winding Pamunkey and took successive supply bases at Eltham's Landing, Cumberland Landing, and finally at White House Landing.[5] This was the point at which the York River Railroad from West Point crossed the Pamunkey to run twenty-three miles straight into Richmond. White House was to be McClellan's base of operations for the final advance on Richmond (Sears 103–104).

Although a relatively small number of men were wounded, an increasing number became sick due to the swampy conditions of the Virginia Peninsula that left water contaminated and typhoid flourishing. Mosquito-borne illnesses weakened soldiers, some of whom were wounded with minie balls and grapeshot, and lack of adequate food and clean water only exacerbated the soldiers' desperate condition. The Sanitary Commission's history describes these days as the "Sisyphus-like movements" of the Army of the Potomac that left "nearly six percent of its force" in hospitals around the Washington, D.C., area (*Works and Purposes* 26). To make matters worse, the same swampy conditions of the battlefield that made men ill also made running a caravan of wagons to transport them virtually impossible. Roads took on the look of "corduroy," as USSC doctors and nurses described them, and the oppressive heat and humidity sapped the strength of even the healthiest of men.

But although overland routes severely impeded the evacuation of sick and wounded soldiers, the rivers and creeks that criss-crossed the peninsula proved life saving. The USSC recognized that the James River, which connected to Chesapeake Bay near Fort Monroe, and the Pamunkey River, accessible via the York River at West Point, as well as the smaller

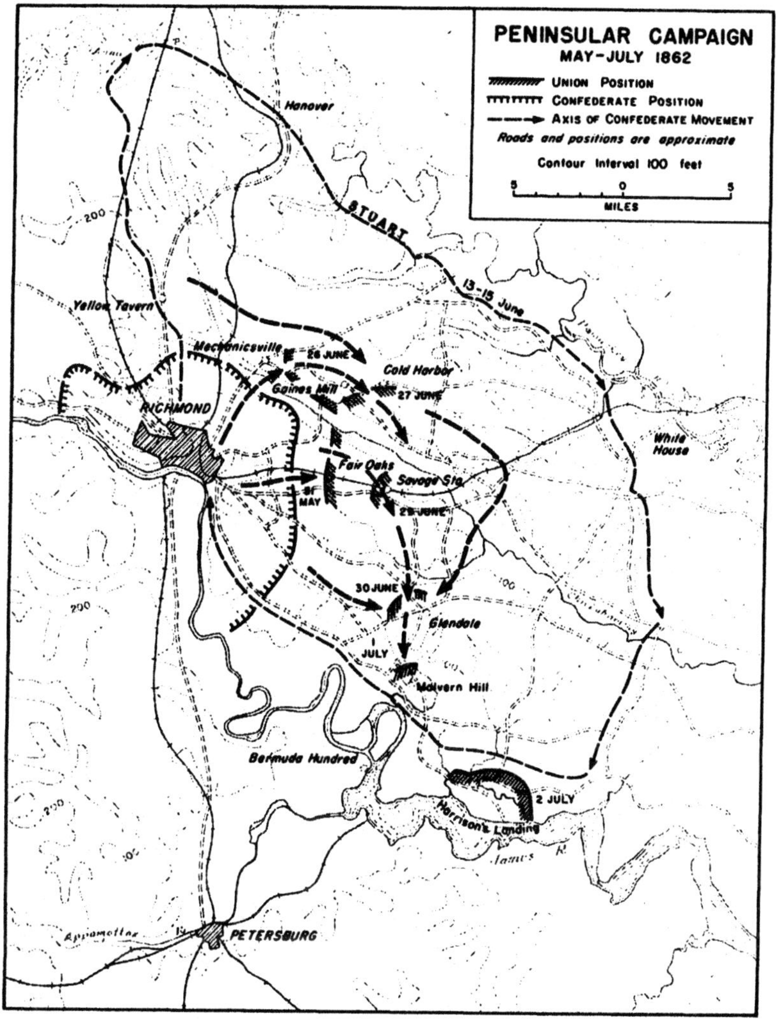

From the Perry Casteñada Library Map Collection at the University of Texas at Austin.

tributaries that split off from these larger rivers, admitted steamers and smaller sailing vessels. The United States Sanitary Commission capitalized on the transport opportunities the rivers presented and requested a number of ships from the government in order to outfit them as hospital transports, complete with USSC surgeons, nurses, and stretcher bearers. McClellan's summer of 1862 campaign of the Virginia Peninsula marked the first time in the war that the hospital transports had been used every day to evacuate and provide floating triage to the Union army (Censer 27).[6]

Throughout the Virginia Campaign, both the Sanitary Commission and the Medical Bureau lacked independent medical transportation, while both employed headstrong physicians and surgeons intent on practicing their best medicine. Although these two distinct groups often worked in harmony with each other, even providing assistance and supplies to each other when needed, the relationship was often contentious. The *Knickerbocker*,[7] for instance, a USSC ship, was anchored off Yorktown one night but the next morning was nowhere to be found, despite searching twice through the fleet. A command had come at midnight, the Sanitary Commission finally learned from the quartermaster's office, and requested that the ship go immediately to the Pamunkey River in advance of the army. The *Knickerbocker* had been sent, one of the women on the hospital ship notes, "the fact of her having been assigned to the Commission being entirely forgotten."

In short, the United States Sanitary Commission too often had its supplies and personnel scrambling to cover simultaneous orders given by multiple offices: the USSC was responsible for military discipline on the ships, the quartermaster had the authority to recall a ship at a moment's notice, military leaders could determine the destination of the transports, and government medical authorities decided where patients should be received and distributed. Frederick Law Olmsted, who was tapped to oversee the USSC's work during the summer of

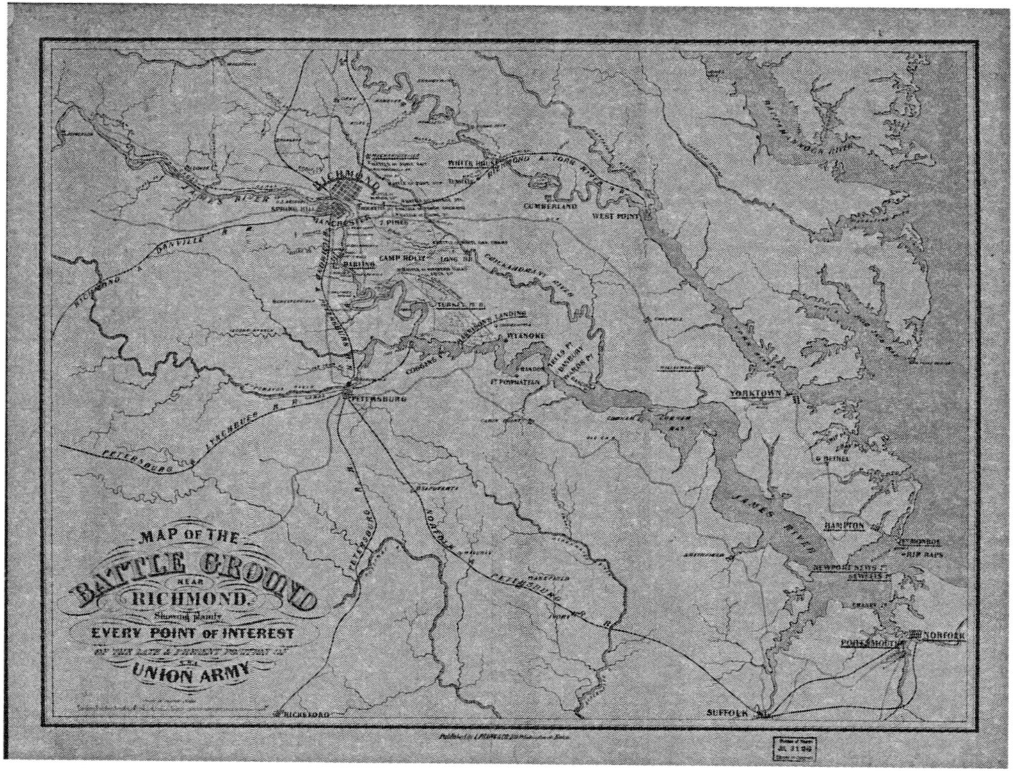

Map of the battle ground near Richmond, showing plainly, every point of interest of the late & present position of the Union Army. L. Prang & Co., Boston, 1862.
From the Library of Congress Geography and Map Division, Washington, D.C.

1862 because of his organizational expertise in public works' projects, "had nine superiors," according to Maxwell. "Each had a different understanding of his duties and problems."

Stretched to their limits, in terms of both supplies and physical and emotional abilities, the transport ships of the Sanitary Commission nonetheless managed to continue their work through the resourcefulness and sheer motivation of their civilian volunteers. "I am quite at a loss to know what I shall do to-morrow," Olmsted confesses in a letter, "Unless additional force arrives we certainly cannot meet another emergency." He then goes on to apologize if his letter "is found somewhat incoherent, for I have fallen asleep several times while writing it." As the summer progressed and the war moved across the peninsula, the tone of the letters becomes increasingly more desperate regarding the lack of supplies, and increasingly more pointed about what the Sanitary Commission perceived was the failure of the U.S. government military corps to tend the sick and wounded. Olmsted complains of having tried "in vain to awaken some of the Headquarters officers to a sense of the danger" that faced them in terms of low supplies and inadequately prepared transport ships. Their reply is rather flippant: "true," Olmsted quotes them in agreement, the wounded "will suffer a good deal for a time, but that is inevitable in war."

The Surgeon General provided no help either, since his office was so overwhelmed with its own responsibilities. In a reply to the Surgeon General, Olmsted suggests that he is ill-equipped to understand that floating hospitals need but "one good authoritative surgeon on board" to keep the organization. He later suggests that "The Surgeon General cannot at once do our sea-transport business as well as we." Yet this was his conclusion after the Sanitary Commission had come to the rescue of yet another government transport ship that claimed to have enough supplies, only to realize once the wounded were being put on board that, in fact, it was desperately low on necessary provisions like food, water, and bandages. "Possibly they have all that is necessary on these government boats, stowed away in boxes somewhere," a nurse writes, "but at the precise moment when it is needed no one knows anything about it. Such boats either have no one at their head, or where there is one there are many, which is worse than none." In short, she concludes, the Sanitary Commission only "seeks to bring the government to do what the government *should* do for its sick and wounded. Until that object is accomplished, the Commission stands ready to throw itself into the breach, as it did during that dreadful battle week, and as it does, more or less, all the time."

To compound these difficulties in sorting through the various chains of command, daily operation of these "Atlantic Floating Hospitals," as Olmsted refers to them, either the USSC's or the Army's fleet, was not easily and efficiently accomplished. Because of the nature of their engagement and the intentions of those on board, they were in a "constant state of preorganization and disorganization." Food was not easy to obtain because of the irregular schedules of supply ships, and once on board, because of the hot and humid weather conditions, fresh food spoiled in a short time. Providing wounded men the proper nourishment also was problematic because of the breaks in the supply chain, and the Sanitary Commission worried about providing a varied diet so as to "avoid the danger of satiety." The sheer number of wounded men to be cared for simultaneously also required that plans of organization and scheduling be quickly made and remade, depending on the situation. "To avoid collisions and vain attempts to perform impossibilities," Olmsted writes, required rules that were not always cheerfully accepted but did provide the structure on which to accomplish their work. He admits in another letter that he "must act a little blindly, sometimes."[8]

The amount of medical supplies that the Sanitary Commission's hospital ships required was enormous; indeed, the numerous battles and small skirmishes between Union and Confederate armies only increased the necessity, not only for these supplies but also for ships to transport the wounded and sick. In a letter to a friend, one of the women volunteers on these ships implores that "I hope people will continue to sustain this great work" of the USSC, most notably its six large vessels now in operation. The "Government furnishes these, and the bare rations of the men, (or is supposed to do so,) but the real expenses of supply fall on the Commission." Then, in an unsolicited request, she tells her friend: "If people ask what they shall send, say, 'Money, *money*, stimulants, and articles of sick-food'."[9] At times, the letters of those who served on the hospital transport ships cease from describing the events of the battlefield or operations of the kitchen in order to comment on the generosity of the Union supporters who continually supplied the commission with money, clothing, and food. "I often wish,—as I give comfort to some poor fellow," a nurse writes, "that the man or woman who supplied the means for the comfort were present to see how blessed it is. Believe me, you may all give and work in the earnest hope that you alleviate suffering, but none of you realize what you do."

"a quantity of letters"

Hospital Transports: A Memoir of the Embarkation of the Sick and Wounded from the Peninsula of Virginia in the Summer of 1862, compiled at the request of the Sanitary Commission by the Woman's Central Army Relief Association of New York, consists of a "quantity of letters and their papers" written by men and women involved in the care and evacuation of the sick and wounded via the hospital transport ships. The letters detail the experiences during the summer of 1862, from the Sanitary Commission's initial outfitting of the *Daniel Webster* on April 30 through the threat of Stonewall Jackson on June 27, 1862, including the Battle of Fair Oaks/Seven Pines in late May and early June. The Woman's Central Army Relief Association selected passages from the letters and compiled this volume in order to "give within moderate compass as many particulars as may be necessary to show the scope of the enterprise, and the position which it held as an aid to the government" (*Hospital Transports* introduction). Several of the letters, although written by various USSC personnel, overlap in their details of events; some were written on the same day but focus on different incidents; still others are undated but are interspersed among letters that carry both dates and locations. This collection was carefully controlled so as to serve as a history to both document and promote the work of the USSC, and inadvertently to provide a record of the military campaigns in Virginia. A review in *The Continental Monthly* remarked on the patriotism of not only the USSC volunteers on the ships, but of the readers; *Hospital Transports* is a book, the review declared, "which should be in the hands of all who love their country" (478). The letters are full of "vivid interest," "true incident," "graphic sketches," and "loyalty, patriotism, and self-abnegation," and as such, provide "succor" for the human race (479). *The Atlantic Monthly* remarked of the USSC that "Wherever the red hand of war is lifted to wound, its white hand may be lifted to heal,—that its work may never cease until it is assumed by a great Christian Government or until peace once more reigns throughout the land" (399).

But more interestingly, *Hospital Transports'* mix of letters provides a rich area for a rhetorical study of the ways that the USSC's male administrators and female nurses narrate their wartime experiences, and how these narratives betray the ideology of benevolence as practiced by upper-middle-class men and women. The volume, however, is complicated because it is a composite memoir, a collection of letters from eight individuals, two officers of the commission and six women serving with them as nurses. Furthermore, the text insists on preserving the anonymity of each author. Individual letters do not bear the name of the author; rather, the Woman's Central Army Relief Association of New York only identified individual writers with alphabet letters: *A* and *B* denote the two male officers, the initials *M* and *N* denote all six of the women. All proper names of the author and audience of the letters have been removed so it is not clear to whom these letters would have been addressed, although, because of the content, many seem to be letters to USSC administration or home. Most references to specific USSC officers and nurses on the transport ships have been removed from within individual letters, as well, although military commanders' names have remained in order to help chart the sequence of events.

Certainly, confidentiality and privacy would have been a concern for the organization charged with compiling these letters. These were personal letters, after all, and provided some level of comfort and intimacy for the men and women working on the hospital ships. Indeed, the relief association admits that those who wrote the letters had "no thought that they could ever go beyond" the friends to whom they were addressed. Moreover, the writers only tell part of the story of their life on the ships, and for the women, the deliberate withholding of experiences provided a means to preserve their jobs, just as the careful editing of the entire collection casts the work of the USSC transport ships in the most impressive possible light. But the anonymity of the writers and the audience also serves to keep the focus entirely on the work of the U.S. Sanitary Commission without personal information, politics, or fame superceding the worthy cause in which the members were engaged. *Hospital Transports* was designed to be a "public record," in the words of the organization that compiled the letters; the whole work of the commission was greater than the sum of its individuals.

What is even more curious, however, is that the letters the six women wrote had to share only two alphabet letters among the six of them. Original readers of *Hospital Transports* were forced to abandon the assumption that in memoir, autobiography, and historical narrative the author is known, and indeed that there even is an author to be recognized. What readers also are asked to abandon, however, is their notion of gendered narratives, gendered work, and social role differences between men and women during the USSC's campaign. Such anonymity, however, only serves to heighten these gender differences in narrative content and approach.

Despite this call to only see the good work of the hospital transport ships during the peninsular campaign, what is evident from the letters of the collection is that men and women were simultaneously engaged in the common act of disciplined care while viewing the war and their responsibilities in far different terms.

Despite the anonymity in *Hospital Transports*, other historical records do reveal who staffed the transport ships during the summer of 1862. Officer *A* is Frederick Law Olmsted; officer *B* is Frederick Newman Knapp, a physician in the USSC. Knapp, ill with malaria, left the Virginia Peninsula around June 11, 1862, to convalesce in his parents' home in Walpole, New Hampshire. The initials *M* and *N* identify letters written by six women on the ships, although, to add to the confusion, at least eight women became permanent members of the transport team: Amy Morris Bradley, Helen Gilson, Christine Kean Griffin, Caroline Lane, Ellen Ruggles Strong, Eliza Woolsey Howland, Georgeanna Woolsey, and Katherine Wormeley. As a result, it is possible to identify only some of the authors of the letters written by women.

Olmsted, who had earned high marks for his planning, development, and administration of New York's Central Park, applied his same organizational acumen to the USSC. He created an administrative regime that allowed quick response to the medical needs of the army wherever it was stationed. The commissioners, Olmsted included, believed that primary responsibility for the care of the soldiers must lie with the Medical Bureau, and thus, they waged a successful campaign to reorganize and expand it and secure a more energetic medical authority (Censer 1). During the period of *Hospital Transports*, Olmsted was present on deck and supervised the hospital ships anchored just off the shore where the Army of the Potomac was camped. According to Jane Turner Censer, Olmsted's greatest achievement with the Sanitary Commission was the "organizational structures emphasizing clearly defined duties, specialization, and the delegation of powers. . . . The combination of a professional staff and tributary local societies provided both an expertise and a flexibility that at the time were nearly unique" (10). In fact, Censer notes, only two other bureaucracies operated with similarly sophisticated systems, the railroad system and the U.S. government (11).

Hospital Transports opens with a letter written by Olmsted dated April 30, 1862, and written on the hospital transport *Daniel Webster, No. 1* in Cheeseman's Creek.[10] The USSC had received the old steamboat on April 25 and Olmsted and Knapp spent the interim days supervising volunteers as they scrubbed the ship from stem to stern, furnished bunks, and outfitted an apothecary's shop. Olmsted's letter details in minute catalog the exact schedule of getting the *Daniel Webster* ready to transport wounded passengers. By Sunday morning, Olmsted writes, the ship's hold was full, by 11 a.m. the hospital company was aboard, but "the commissaries failed in their engagements" and he had to send a foraging party to Alexandria for beef. At 4 p.m. the meat had been put on board and "we at once got under way." Olmsted then provides a list of the initial passengers: six medical students, twenty volunteer male nurses, four surgeons, four ladies, a dozen "contrabands" described as "field hands," three carpenters, and six miscellaneous passengers. Five members of the U.S. Sanitary Commission were also aboard, as were eight military officers, ninety soldiers returning to their regiments, several mechanics, and the ship's crew and officers.

On May 1, Knapp writes that they had joined other commission boats, one or two storeships and, notably, the *Wilson Small*, anchored off Shipping Point. The area had once been controlled by the Confederate army, but now the Union used it for a hospital. The *Wilson Small*[11] was a small light boat that had been outfitted as a "little hospital, to run up creeks and bring down sick and wounded to the transports." Throughout *Hospital Transports*, the *Wilson Small* can be followed darting in and out of shallow tributaries and creeks, loading up with wounded soldiers, and then delivering them to the larger, heavier transport ships that would then ferry them to the field hospitals on and up the coast. The *Daniel Webster* received its first patients in just this way.

While it was dark, the *Wilson Small* came alongside the *Daniel Webster*, carrying thirty-five wounded soldiers. They were carefully lifted on board and "swung through the hatches on their stretchers." Within thirty minutes, the soldiers had all been given tea or coffee by the nurses, then shortly afterward were undressed and put to bed clean and comfortable; the men, one of the nurses remarked, were "in a droll state of grateful wonder." By May 3, 190 patients had come aboard the *Daniel Webster* and even more had been treated on shore by Sanitary Commission surgeons and nurses who offered their services at the Ship's Point Hospital.

Hospital Transports continues with this complex description of the work the transport ships did during the peninsular campaign. The two officers, *A* (Olmsted) and *B* (Knapp), categorize the intricate workings of the ships, their personnel, and the political tension that existed between the federal government's medical corps and the U.S. Sanitary Commission. *A* and *B* count surgeons and men, discuss the daily outfitting and operating techniques of running floating hospitals, and tell the exploits of securing beef for one ship, and cotton gauze for another. In short, their letters are the stories of administrators engaged in running an efficient and smooth operation.

Yet the presence of women on the ships represented a departure from the USSC's policy, even though Dr. Elizabeth Blackwell's Women's Central Association of Relief (WCAR) original proposal was to recruit, train, and assign a corps of nurses to assist with the war effort in an effort to "bring order from the supposed chaos of benevolent enthusiasm" (Ginzberg 141). The young women involved in relief work "expressed a new elitism," Ginzberg avers, "one that rejected the tenets of 'virtuous femininity' that had characterized the antebellum era—and to which most women still adhered" (144). But even before Olmsted and Bellows were recruited, the Women's Central Association of Relief, the precursor to the New York organization and headed by Dr. Elizabeth Blackwell, proposed to assign a corps of trained women nurses to the commission. When Olmsted and Bellows took the plan to Washington, D.C., however, "they largely abandoned the issues of nurses" (Giesberg 115) since they were more interested in establishing the credibility of the commission, a task that pushed the issue of trained nurses out of primary attention and reinforced the army's resistance to allowing women on the battlefield and in the field hospitals.

Olmsted, however, recognized that women's presence on the ships would allow him "to tap into the domestic rhetoric of the middle-class home," Giesberg suggests, "a strategy that had worked well to garner support for his work on Central Park" (123). He had effectively promoted the park as "a separate sphere of the middle-class home" and a "healing environment." The hospital transports ships were, for Olmsted, "an experiment in bringing the home to the battlefield" and he recruited middle-class and elite women to serve as nurses. What united the USSC commissioners and these women was the assumption about "the proper role" these "lady volunteers" were to occupy on the ships, and the experiences they brought with them, namely, their "familiarity with genteel standards of household organization" (Ross 100, 101). Indeed, one of the women serving on the transports declares that she looks forward to the return of the *Wilson Small* so that they can "resume our happy *home* life on the top of the old stove."

If *Hospital Transports* is a complicated collection of letters because of the deliberate anonymity assigned to its writers, then the nature of the USSC work on the ships is even more complex. The nineteenth century witnessed great changes in the conception of voluntarism as a means for not only social good, but social improvements. The Second Great Awakening (late 1820s to early 1830s) and the formation of the Women's Christian Temperance Union in 1874 bookend the formation of the ladies' aid societies formed to provide for soldiers in the Civil War. In providing this altruistic service, Giesberg argues that the USSC served as an "interim structure for women's activism" (11). In doing so,

Giesberg continues, these women "created a new political culture for women" that combined "grassroots activism with centralized access to political authority" (8).

In order to occupy such a nationally political transitional state, the personal politics of the women had to adapt. Much has been made of what historians have called "the cult of true womanhood" and the assumed "true morality" they possessed. "As long as woman did not leave her sphere [her home]," Ginzberg explains, "God had ordained that she be protected by some inherent goodness, a 'moral organ' in her very being" (11). Yet the supposition that there even was a "woman's sphere" was a particularly middle- and upper-middle-class philosophy, one that becomes even more complicated given the ideology of "benevolence" that pervaded middle- and late-nineteenth-century American society. Women's morality manifested itself in charitable acts, or "benevolence," and women described such work as Christian, "their means as fundamentally moral, and their mandate as uniquely female" (Ginzberg 1). Yet, as Ginzberg quickly points out, the ideology of "women's sphere" was only a superficial way of linking women together, even within the middle class. Conservative benevolent women, Ginzberg claims, "were far more likely than abolitionists to be members of wealthy, locally influential family and community networks, and their benevolent goals and means reflected the economic and political privileges of their class" (Ginzberg 6).

The women who served on the hospital ships, whose letters are included in *Hospital Transports* labeled by the initials *M* and *N*, suggest not only this politically gendered bias that women were ideally suited and indeed expected to cook and care for others, but represent the specific class-based ideology of the USSC since they were drawn from the same class and social status as the officers and physicians (Ross 100). According to an article in the *Sanitary Commission Bulletin*, "The women [on the transport ships] belong nearly all to the most wealthy or most respectable families." The *Bulletin* expressed pleasant surprise with their successful service since "it could not be supposed that their former habits of comfort and luxury could prepare them for encountering the perils and privations which they must necessarily meet with in this field of labor" (in Ginzberg 147–48).

Katherine Wormeley, for example, organized volunteers to make army shirts when the Civil War began; during the winter of 1861–62, she sold the fifty thousand shirts to the quartermaster of the Army (for about $6,000) and distributed the money to needy families of soldiers. In May, 1862, she volunteered for duty with the Sanitary Commission in Virginia as a superintendent of nursing, and left the Virginia Peninsula in July 1862. Georgeanna Muirson Woolsey and Eliza Newton Woolsey Howland were sisters, two of the eight Woolsey women (and one son) to serve in the Civil War. Despite the death of their father at an early age, the Woolsey children and their mother, Jane, of Eight Brevoort Place in New York City, were wealthy, better educated than most women of their day, and were strongly abolitionist. Georgeanna, nicknamed "Georgie," was one of the first women trained under the program of the Women's Central Association of Relief, under the direction of Dr. Elizabeth Blackwell. Eliza was trained as a nurse before serving on the transport ships and was a nurse at the Patent Office Hospital in Washington. And, as Agatha Young records, Eliza, Georgeanna, and all of the women of the Woolsey family attended the final meeting of the Women's Central Relief Association in New York City (382).

Other women, such as Christine Griffin[12] and Eliza Harris, both early volunteers with the transport service during the Virginia Peninsula campaign, came from this particular upper-class section of American society. Early in the war, Harris oversaw the army relief funds from Pennsylvania and later took charge of the service for the wounded at Fortress Monroe (Greenbie 133). A prolific fundraiser, Harris wrote dramatic accounts to newspapers detailing her life aboard the ships, including special references to all the supplies the transport ships were lacking. After the Battle of Fair Oaks/Seven Pines she writes that "There were 800 on board.

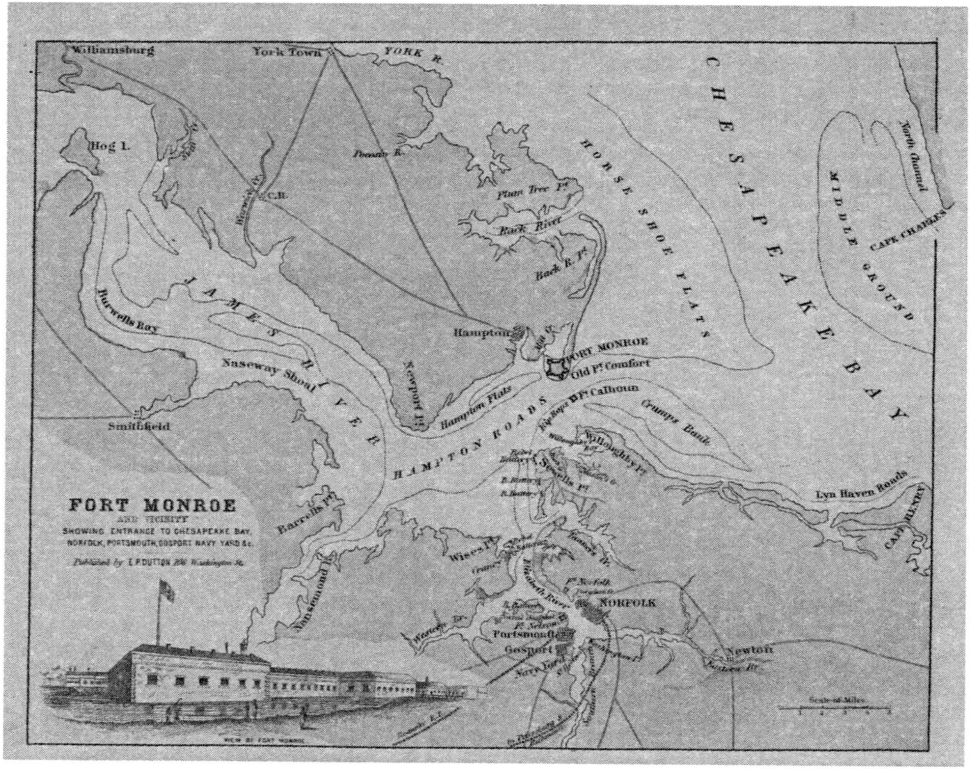

Fort Monroe and vicinity showing entrance to Chesapeake Bay, Norfolk, Portsmouth, Gosport Navy Yard &c. Boston, 186–. From the Library of Congress Geography and Map Division, Washington D.C.

Passage-ways, state-rooms, floors, from the dark and foetid hold to the hurricane deck, were more than filled—some of the wounded on mattresses, others on straw; some in the death struggle, others nearing it, some in their blood as they had been brought from the battle-field of the Sabbath previous, and all hungry and thirsty." As Marjorie Barstow Greenbie notes, "Readers of such a story would hurry off money, supplies, and workers in the next boat for 'poor dear Mrs. Harris' " (133). But although the USSC's own publication expressed surprise at "respectable" women's successes on the transports, it was precisely their class status, and the ideologies that were embedded in it, that allowed these women to imagine, participate in, and ultimately change medical care during the Civil War. Giesberg explains that the young women of the USSC "drew on common traditions of women's culture and preserved the sex-segregated autonomy of women's local grassroots activism. At the same time, however, they imagined themselves and their interests as part of an extended women's community that transcended local interests and the borders of towns and states" (7).

Transport women's work, however, was even more complex than this careful negotiaton between local and national gendered politics. Although some of the women, such as the Woolsey sisters, had been trained as nurses, many of the women lacked formal training, but all entered with two key attributes particular to their class and background, according to Kristie Ross: "an eagerness to seize an occasion to escape the routine pattern of their lives and a familiarity with genteel standards of household organization" (101), namely order, efficiency, foresight, and an appreciation of cleanliness (104). Ginzberg concurs, suggesting that "nationalism, discipline, centralization, and, above all, efficiency became the watchwords of a new benevolence" (133), one that differed markedly from the ideologies of an earlier era that relied on individual moral perfection. In essence, they placed benevolent work "on a corporate footing" and "proposed that scientific rather than moral principles characterize social welfare" (Ginzberg 134). In short, as Ginzberg notes, the legacy of the USSC was "an elitist repudiation of an older style of female benevolence" (172).

The second letter of *Hospital Transports* provides a marked contrast to the letters written by Olmsted and Knapp. Written by one of the women given the initial *M*, this account bears no date or geographic locator although, given its placement, it presumably also details the events on the *Daniel Webster*'s first voyage to Cheeseman's Creek. Like Olmsted's letter, *M* also catalogs how the time was spent, although her letter describes the women's activities. Since it was the Sabbath, these women put together a makeshift church service on the deck of the ship with a chaplain offering what *M* terms an " 'unprepared' discourse upon charity." Honoring the importance of Sunday worship while at the same time understanding their mission on the transport ship, the women sang hymns while they engaged in the "secular occupation" of sewing a large hospital flag. Finally, *M* makes special note of the "singing of the contrabands, who all came in and stood in a row so black, at the dark end of the cabin, that I could see neither eyes nor teeth. But they sung heartily," *M* notes, "and everybody followed them."

The women, of course, were administrators of a different sort in the U.S. Sanitary Commission, and exercised their control over domestic responsibilities. They were intent on showing their support for the Union soldiers by being their caretakers, surrogate mothers or sisters or wives, at least for the short time they were being transported from battlefield to hospital via ship. Their letters are, not surprisingly given gender roles and stereotypes, concerned with the operations of the kitchen and mess, the sad stories of young soldiers, and the human camaraderie that would naturally arise when people work in such close quarters for a prolonged period of time.[13] The ongoing war even seems secondary, at times, in the ladies' letters; what replaces it is the insistence that they are successfully nursing the soldiers who are in need of efficiently distributed comfort. The women arranged for prayers to be read for the whole company, the crew and the soldiers. They handed out clean clothes, handkerchiefs, and cologne, and served dinner according to the diet prescribed for each soldier's injury or illness. As Ross explains, these "female superintendent [s] were assigned to duty by Olmsted where he felt they were most needed and frequently arranged their own hours of rotation," depending on the needs of each transport ship (101). "The house-diet, which was all distributed from our pantry," *M* describes with pride, "was nice thick soup and rice-pudding, and we made over our spirit-lamps, the beef-tea and gruels for special cases." Days ended with the ladies sitting in the pantry and "talking over evils to be remedied," according to *M*, such as "should the soiled clothes be sewed up in canvas-bags and trailed behind the ship, or hung at the stern, or headed up in barrels and steam-washed when the ship got in?"

The seemingly mundane chores of the women seem to pale against the political strife happening in the divided country. Yet matters of hygiene and sustenance for wounded or dying soldiers were clearly life-and-death issues as well, as these women keenly realized. Unable to take up arms and march with regiments against the Confederates, this hospital work was their vital contribution to the Union. It is not surprising, then, that Georgeanna Woolsey (*M*) should write matter-of-factly: "While we were lying anchored off Ship Point, down in the Gulf, New Orleans had surrendered quietly, and round the corner from us Fort Macon had been taken. What was it all to us, so long as the beef-tea was ready at the right moment?"

It is clear that the "great work" of the Sanitary Commission's hospital transports clearly could not have succeeded or even continued without the "ladies" on the ships. But what is also striking is that the "great work" by women who volunteered for hospital duty on these ships changed the women by presenting them with a markedly freer atmosphere on these transports that allowed them experiences they never would have been allowed to have on land; their work on the ships, as Giesberg notes, did not replicate the middle-class domestic relations from which they had come (120). As the battle on the Virginia Peninsula progressed through the summer, these hospitals became a kind of floating island, distanced literally from the land, but more importantly, distanced metaphorically from the stereotyped expectations that governed women's behavior. The horrific events of the campaign, in short, allowed these women to renegotiate their gendered status and to adapt their behaviors.

The ladies "are just what they should be," Katherine Wormeley (*N*) writes, "efficient, wise, active as cats, merry, lighthearted, thoroughbred, and without the fearful tone of self-devotedness about them that sad experience makes one expect in benevolent women." Olmsted (*A*) remarks that the ladies are a "great godsend" who "worked like heroes night and day" often doing work that is "frequently of the most disagreeable and trying character." Yet, he proudly notes, "I have never seen one of them flinch for a moment." The women's response is, perhaps, most telling. Rather than lamenting on the difficulty of the work or about the unsanitary and public conditions on board the ships, one of the women, *M*, replies: "I never had half the present satisfaction in any week of my life before!" and, Olmsted (*A*) notes, "there was a general murmur of concurrence."

The freedom the hospital transport ships permitted the women in their exercise of gender "highlighted the artificiality and socially contrived nature of the symbols and assigned attributes of gender," Ross writes (105). For the weeks they served on the ships, the men and the women put aside their genderings to focus solely on ministering to the sick and horribly wounded without losing their faith in order and discipline. Georgeanna Woolsey, acutely aware of her surroundings, marvels to her mother how strange it is "that the sight of such misery, such death in life, should have been accepted by us all so quietly as it was" (from Ross 108). Even Olmsted remarks on the psychological strength of the women in the face of horror. After the Battle of Fair Oaks/Seven Pines, he explains, soldiers "arrived, dead and living together, in the same close box, many with awful wounds festering and swarming with maggots. Recollect it was midsummer in Virginia, clear and calm. The stench was such as to produce vomiting with some of our strong men. . . . Need I tell you," he continues, "that the women were always ready to press into these places of horror, going to them in torrents of rain, groping their way by dim lantern light, at all hours of night?"

Yet despite the loosening of these restrictions, "neither the women nor their male colleagues were necessarily encouraged by the complexity of what they saw" (Ross 105), nor could they articulate fully the gendered behavior they witnessed. Forty "Sisters" had arrived on the peninsula unexpectedly, but instead of helping the USSC nurses, they "had all struck for keys to their staterooms, and sat about on their large trunks, forbidden to stir by the Padre, who was in a high state of ecclesiastical disgust on the deck of the *Knickerbocker*." The "Sisters" remained "fastened to their places by the Padre's eyes," as one of the nurses writes, "and not one of them was allowed to come over and help us." Yet when the women on board make sense of this episode, they do so in the language of benevolent discipline, rather than reading the "Sisters'" inability to act without the Padre's approval as a sign of strict gendered behavior: "It is unpleasant," one nurse comments, "to abuse people for inefficiency." These women did not so much enlarge their sphere of influence during the Civil War as Olmsted notes, the care of the wounded was "not a feminine business," but instead "It must have a masculine discipline" (from Attie 55). Instead, they changed its venue by bringing "home" to the wounded men on the hospital transport ships.

The pattern of a woman's letter followed or preceded by a letter from Olmsted or Knapp reveals the carefully gendered space of the narrative as a whole, as do the two alphabet letters attached to six individual's correspondence. Throughout *Hospital Transports*, the women whose letters were identified by *M* and *N* are forced to share space with Olmsted (*A*), and through careful editing, their experiences are clearly proscribed to adhere to the rhetoric of upper-class benevolence. The women's letters have been deliberately edited to speak only of their cooking and cleaning acumen, their efficient organization of the beds and men, while their complaints are registered in the tenor of *M,* who reports that the commission performed its work as best it could, not from any mandate. As one example of these terrible conditions, *M* reports that there was not even a cup or a pail to distribute food, "if there had been any provisions in the first place."

The Woman's Central Army Relief Association of New York's completed composition of *Hospital Transports* is, finally, a remarkably complex, sociopolitical text. Olmsted's insistence on maintaining the gendered relations of the genteel home was replicated not only on the boats but also in the completed manuscript. If *Hospital Transports* is considered a documentary of the USSC's success during the Virginia campaign, it also must be understood as propaganda, not only explicitly as a way to promote the commission's medical expertise, but implicitly, by its careful inclusion of only certain letters by transport ship personnel, for its reinforcement of distinct male and female spheres of influence and experience and the way USSC provided male control over female enthusiasm (Ginzberg 173). As such, *Hospital Transports* provides an important marketing tool for the Woman's Central Army Relief Association: the women on the hospital ships had clearly proven their worth to the USSC, their letters home to their families, detailing their competency and successes, were proof that women should continue to be involved in the war effort, and even more so, that an organized benevolence provided unsurpassed care.

The narrative of the Sanitary Commission's hospital transports ends with the ships, medical personnel, and remaining troops being commanded to hurriedly retreat, out of the rivers and streams and back up the coast to Harrison's Landing. Stonewall Jackson was threatening raids against the hospitals since they were so well equipped with much needed medical supplies, and the Confederate army was making a

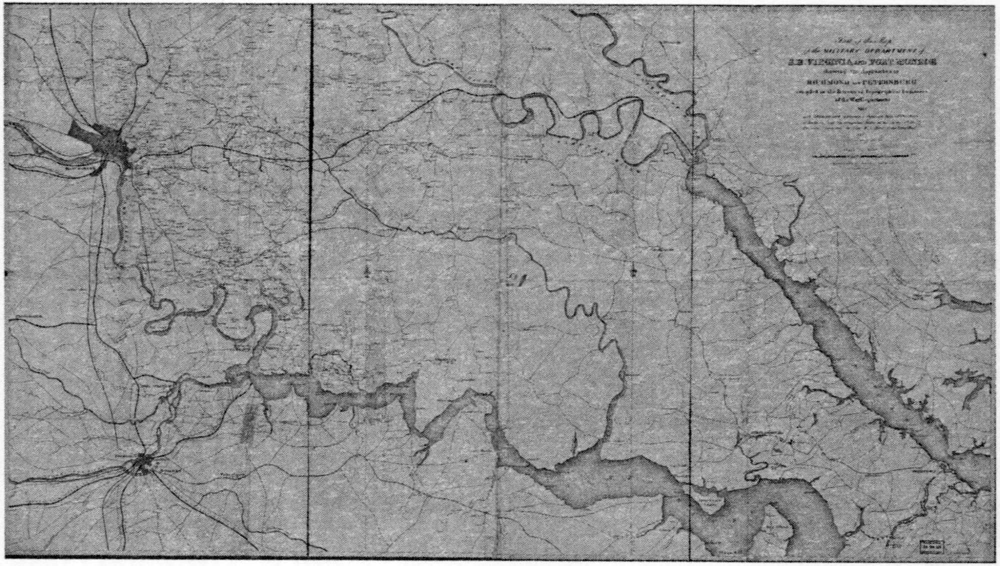

Part of the map of the military department of S.E. Virginia and Fort Monroe, showing the approaches to Richmond and Petersburg compiled in the Bureau of Topographical Engineers of the War Department, 1861, with additions and corrections from the map of the siege of Yorktown and the campaign maps of the Army of the Potomac, compiled by Capt. H. L. Abbot, Corps Topolgl. Engrs. Engraved on stone by J. Schedler, 1862.

From the Library of Congress Geography and Map Division, Washington, D.C.

push toward White House. On June 26, Olmsted received notice that the Sanitary Commission was to leave White House by evening since Confederate troops had seized the railroad and cut the telegraph wire. As the commission's transports pulled away from the shore, Olmsted describes that when it became known to the slaves that, as he phrases it, "the Yankees were running away," they came flocking to the shore carrying their possessions, hoping to be taken aboard the ships. Fortunately, he writes, there was plenty of room on the decks of the forage boats and the men, women, and children climbed on board. "The day of deliverance had come," he announces, "and they accepted this most wonderful change in absolute placidity," quietly nursing their children and singing.

Hospital Transports ultimately describes not only important historical moments in the Civil War, the Virginia Peninsula, and the United States Sanitary Commission. It also reveals a changing attitude by its "lady volunteers," what Ross describes as a "subtle undermining of bourgeois gender distinctions" (98). They entered the ships' hospital service because of their genteel domesticity and left the ships, some only a scant three months later, fully self-confident in their own abilities, brimming with new skills, and mindful of the terrible carnage to which they had been exposed. But although the Sanitary Commission's work on the Virginia Peninsula had accomplished much, it left the men and women of the USSC transport service frustrated. As the *Wilson Small* slowly pulled away amid the increasing frequency of fire-flashes over the trees toward White House, Olmsted recounts the USSC's work in those past eleven weeks, running its ships back and forth from the shore to Fortress Monroe, Washington, and Boston, carrying thousands of sick and wounded soldiers. They came to think of that place as "a sort of home," Olmsted remarks, "where we had all worked together and been happy." He was disheartened, however, by the continued disorganization and conflicting authority between the army's Medical Bureau and the USSC. "Never did Olmsted find the Sanitary Commission's position to be more anomalous or more open to conflicting interpretation," according to Censer (31). He could do little more than offer mixed reviews of the USSC's work in their hospital transport campaign.[14] In a letter to Henry Bellows on July 13, 1862, Olmsted writes: "This summer's work had paid splendidly in lives saved and pain alleviated; it is valuable (sic) also negatively as indicating what our function is not. But as to improving the service—upon my conscience, I believe the average transport service would be better than it is, if we had never touched it" (Censer 405).

Despite Olmsted's assessment, the U.S. Sanitary Commission had succeeded despite terrible environmental conditions and the disorganization of the federal government's medical corps. Its work during the summer of 1862 was vitally important in supporting the Union troops and instigating organizational plans for personnel movements on a similarly large scale. Most specifically, the commission remained true to its original goal, clearly articulated by one of its many volunteers: the Sanitary Commission "seeks to bring the government to do what the government *should* do for its sick and wounded." Although there were rumors that this change should soon be effected, "the officers and nurses of the Sanitary Commission did not let the rumor of change affect their work." "If pure benevolence was ever organized and utilized into beneficence," *The Atlantic Monthly* waxed, "the name of the institution is the Sanitary Commission" and it remained committed to the "great work" of caring for the sick and wounded, on land and water.

Notes

1. George Brinton McClellan was hailed at the beginning of the war as the "Young Napoleon." He proved to be a brilliant military organizer, administrator, and trainer of men but an officer totally lacking in the essential qualities of the successful command of large forces in battle. Given command of the armies around Washington (Div. of the Potomac) and later succeeding General

Scott, he undertook with marked success the complex task of organizing and training the Union armies. His failure in the peninsular campaign led Halleck to give Pope command of the next major operation. After the latter's defeat at the second Battle of Bull Run, McClellan resumed his former role. The administration became increasingly dissatisfied with his reluctance to march against the enemy. After Antietam, when McClellan delayed in pursuing Lee, Lincoln finally lost patience and ordered Burnside to take command of the Army of the Potomac.

2. Charles Stuart Tripler served as medical director of the Army of the Potomac from August 1861 to June 1862. A graduate of the College of Physicians and Surgeons, he received his commission as an army surgeon in 1830. Dr. Jonathan Letterman replaced Tripler as medical director on July 3, 1862.

3. The *Daniel Webster No. 2* was built in 1853 or 1854, it was smaller than the other side-wheeled steamer, the *Daniel Webster No. 1*.

4. In May 1861 at Fortress Monroe, Virginia, General Benjamin F. Butler decided not to return runaway slaves to disloyal masters but to designate then "contraband of war" and set them to work in Union camps (Censer 4).

5. White House was the Custis family plantation which, during the Civil War, belonged to William Henry Fitzhugh "Rooney" Lee, one of Robert E. Lee's sons. One hundred years earlier, White House had been the site of George Washington's courtship of the widow Martha Custis. General Lee's wife was a Custis and had been staying at White House just a few days before the Union army had come (Sears 104).

6. Not only did this floating ambulance service provide an opportunity for the men of the USSC to serve the army, but as Giesberg argues, it also was "a unique opportunity to promote the organization. By stopping to help the U.S. Army as it went further into the South," she writes, "the commission proved once again that it was prepared to take on any new challenge the war presented and that commission men were organization experts whose contributions were integral to the success of the Union war effort" (114).

7. The *Knickerbocker* was an 858-ton steamboat built in New York in 1843. According to Olmsted, the *Knickerbocker* "is a very old boat, low between decks and in the hull, with no means of ventilation under the main deck and consequently of scarcely

more than half the capacity of other boats of not much greater length and with which she would by a careless observer be classed."

8. Intent on precisely detailing their organizational benevolence, *Hospital Transports* contains two appendices that specify the exact amount and type of food given to soldiers, as well as the number of patients each transport ship could transport to the hospital from the staging area at White House.

9. This blunt request for funds to enable the Sanitary Commission's continued work might have been a direct result of the little press coverage they received. Maxwell writes that Olmsted complained that newspaper correspondents "were all at the front but showed little care for the dispositions of the sick as did the generals." How were the people to learn about floating hospitals, he wondered, especially since the undertaking seemed too expensive and too vast for private resources (149).

10. The *Daniel Webster No. 1,* according to the quartermaster's report, was "an old Pacific steamer of small capacity." It was assigned to the USSC on April 27; on May 2, it received its first patients, 32 sick soldiers from Ship Point Hospital. Soon after, the total cargo reached 184 patients.

11. The *Wilson Small* was a side-wheeled steamboat built in 1851 and weighing 258 tons. Workers in the USSC renamed it the *Collida* because it was so often struck and damaged by other ships in the harbor (Censer 332 n. 1).

12. Christine Kean Griffin (c. 1826–1915), widow of naval officer William Preston Griffin, served on the Board of Managers of the Women's Central Association of Relief. She served as a superintendent on the the transport ships from early May 1862 until illness forced her to return to New York on June 19. In less than a month she returned to her work on the hospital ships. Katherine P. Wormeley believed Griffin combined efficiency with great aplomb and abilities and described her as a "magnificent" worker. Olmsted, too, admired her abilities. When he drew up a plan to stimulate army enlistments by hiring female store clerks to replace young males who could then enlist, he first submitted it to her for advice.

13. See Judith Ann Giesberg's book, *Civil War Sisterhood: The U.S. Sanitary Commission and Women's Politics in Transition*, for a more in-depth discussion of the vital role of women in the development, organization, and implementation of the USSC.

14. Olmsted relinquished his post in the field and sailed to New York on July 16, 1862. In late July 1862, Olmsted returned to supervising Sanitary Commission affairs in Washington; in the fall of 1863, he resigned from the commission.

References

Attie, Jeanie. *Patriotic Toil: Northern Women and the American Civil War*. Ithaca, NY: Cornell University Press, 1998.

Censer, Jane Turner, editor. *Defending the Union: The Civil War and the U.S. Sanitary Commission, 1961–1863. The Papers of Frederick Law Olmsted* v.4. Baltimore: Johns Hopkins University Press, 1986.

"Sanitary Commission No. 1, An Address to the Secretary of War." *Documents of the U.S. Sanitary Commission*. Number 1–60. New York, 1866.

Giesberg, Judith Ann. *Civil War Sisterhood: The U.S. Sanitary Commission and Women's Politics in Transition*. Boston: Northeastern University Press, 2000.

Ginzberg, Lori D. *Women and the Work of Benevolence: Morality, Politics, and Class in the Nineteenth-Century United States*. New Haven, Conn.: Yale University Press, 1990.

Greenbie, Marjorie Barstow. *Lincoln's Daughters of Mercy*. New York: Putnam, 1944.

Hospital Transports: A Memoir of the Embarkation of the Sick and Wounded from the Peninsula of Virginia in the Summer of 1862. Boston: Ticknor and Fields, 1863.

Maxwell, William Quentin. *Lincoln's Fifth Wheel: The Political History of the United States Sanitary Commission*. New York: Longmans, Green, 1956.

McPherson, James M. *Ordeal by Fire: The Civil War and Reconstruction*. Third edition. New York: Mc-Graw Hill, 2001.

"Peninsular Campaign, May–July 1862." Map. From the Perry-Castañeda Library Map Collection, University of Texas at Austin.

Rev. of *Hospital Transports. The Atlantic Monthly*, v. XII (September 1863): 398–99.

Rev. of *Hospital Transports. The Continental Monthly*, v. IV (July–December 1863): 478–79.

Ross, Kristie. "Arranging a Doll's House: Refined Women as Union Nurses." *Divided Houses: Gender and the Civil War*. Edited by Catherine Clinton and Nina Silber. New York: Oxford University Press, 1992.

The Sanitary Commission of the United States Army: A Succinct Narrative of Its Works and Purposes. 1864. New York: Arno Press and *New York Times,* 1972.

Sears, Stephen W. *To the Gates of Richmond: The Peninsula Campaign*. New York: Ticknor and Fields, 1992.

Wormeley, Katharine Prescott. *The Other Side of War with the Army of the Potomac*. Boston: Ticknor, 1889.

Young, Agatha. *The Women and the Crisis: Women of the North in the Civil War*. New York: McDowell, Obolensky, 1959.

Part Two

Hospital Transports.

Hospital Transports.

A Memoir

of the

EMBARKATION OF THE SICK AND WOUNDED FROM THE PENINSULA OF VIRGINIA IN THE SUMMER OF 1862.

Compiled and Published at the request of the Sanitary Commission.

Boston:
Ticknor and Fields.
1863.

UNIVERSITY PRESS:
WELCH, BIGELOW, AND COMPANY,
Cambridge.

Dedication.

TO THE MEMORIES OF

J. M. GRYMES, M.D.,
sometime Surgeon in charge of the Hospital Transport *Daniel Webster*, and, at the time of his death, Surgeon to the temporary *Home* for disabled soldiers, of the Sanitary Commission at Washington;—

WILLIAM PLATT, JUNIOR, ESQ.,
late a Relief Agent of the Sanitary Commission, who died from the effect of prolonged exposure and excessive exertion in pushing succor to the wounded during and after the battles of South Mountain, Crampton's Gap, and Antietam;—

Lieut.-Col. JOSEPH BRIDGHAM CURTIS, U.S.V.,
formerly of the Engineer Corps of the Central Park of New York, afterwards of the central staff of the Sanitary Commission, who fell while leading his regiment to the assault of the rebel works at Fredericksburg, December, 1862;—

RUDD C. HOPKINS, M.D.,
formerly Superintendent of the Lunatic Asylum of Ohio, lately a General Inspector of the Sanitary Commission, and who died in its service, while on the river passage from Memphis to Cincinnati;—

MRS. FANNY SWAN WARRINER,
who bore heroically to the end a woman's part in war, having died at Louisville, Kentucky, on her way home from the Head-quarters Relief Station of the Sanitary Commission with the Army of the Tennessee,—of disease there contracted;—

DAVID BOSWELL REID, M.D.,
Fellow of the Royal Society of Edinburgh; Fellow of the Royal College of Physicians of London; Member of the Medico-Chirurgical Society of St. Petersburg; formerly Director of Ventilation at the Houses of Parliament of Great Britain; late Professor of Physiology and Hygiene at the University of Wisconsin; at the time of his death, Special Inspector of the Ventilation of Hospitals of the Sanitary Commission;—and

Surgeon ROBERT WARE, U.S.V.,
for several years physician in charge of the largest Dispensary District in Boston, afterwards a General Inspector of the Sanitary Commission, and Surgeon of its Relief Stations at Yorktown, White House, and Berkeley, lastly Surgeon of Volunteers. He fell at his post in the works at Washington, North Carolina, during its bombardment by the rebels, March, 1863.

Introduction

The Sanitary Commission, grateful for the generous confidence reposed in it by the public, would be glad to meet and justify that confidence by a circumstantial account of its operations in field and hospital, from the first day of its existence to the present. It might, perhaps, without undue boasting, show such a picture of what has been accomplished as would stimulate, to the last degree, the interest and the liberality of loyal hearts, if this were required. But the immense mass of details which such an account must involve, would prove nearly as laborious in the reading as in the performance, overwhelming rather than enlightening all who have not been personally engaged in the work. The intense interest which the service inspires in those devoted to it, lightens what might, under other circumstances, seem wearisome duties; but a minute description of the ceaseless round of consultations, examinations, correspondence, journeys, accounts, distributions, required of the Commission as trustee of the public bounty, could not be expected to prove interesting to others.

The most that the Commission can at present be called upon to offer, or the public be likely to accept, is such brief accounts of single sections in the various departments of its labor, as may indicate the general method and spirit extending through the whole. In accordance with this plan, from time to time, the Commission has published reports covering a single battle-field, or a term of one round of visits to the hospitals, or the results of its arrangements for the care of disabled and discharged soldiers for a stated period. There is one branch of the service, however, which has as yet had no such public record,—that of the Hospital Transports. In order to supply this omission in some measure, the Commission has caused to be placed in the hands of a manager of the "Woman's Central Army Relief Association of New York," a quantity of letters and other papers, containing observations made at the time, and on the spot, by those in its service who assisted in the embarkation and care of the sick and wounded on the peninsula of Virginia in 1862. Passages from these have been selected and arranged with a view to give within moderate compass as many particulars as may be necessary to show the scope of the enterprise, and the position which it held as an aid to the government, together with the difficulties and the success, the disappointments and satisfactions, with which it was attended. The plan is limited to the Atlantic hospital transports, and to the period of embarkation of the patients upon them, for the sake of compactness and completeness in the grouping of incidents. A similar service in the Western rivers the same year was larger in its scope, and in some of its arrangements more satisfactory, but it was at the same time less homogeneous in character.

For the style of the letters quoted, this only need be said: they were, for the most part, addressed to intimate friends, with no thought that they could ever go beyond them, or, as in the case of those addressed by the Secretary to the President of the Commission, were in the nature of familiar and confidential reports; nearly all were written hastily, in some chance interruption to severe labor,—often with a pencil, while passing in a boat from one vessel to another. Passages may be found which are not merely descriptive of the Hospital Transport service, but they contain thoughts springing from the occasion, and which will serve to fasten pictures of scenes and circumstances with which that service was associated, and which are now historical.*

It should be understood that the account is not intended to be complete in any respect, and that no attempt has been made to give public credit to individuals for their services, whatever these may have been. It is known that to do so in some cases where public gratitude is most deserved would give pain; to do so in all cases would greatly swell the bulk of the volume. In general terms only it may be said, that among the surgeons who freely gave their aid in the enterprise were numbered some of the leading members of the profession,—among those who served as administrative officers, matrons, and nurses, the most honored historical families of New England, New York, New Jersey, and Pennsylvania were represented. The class termed Ward-masters was mainly composed of medical students of two years, with some young men of Philadelphia who had had previous experience in caring for sick soldiers in the noble local charities of that city. It included, also, some students of theology. The responsibility for the detail of care of the patients was chiefly with this class, and the devotedness, pliability, and practical talent with which they generally met this responsibility was too remarkable to be passed without at least this simple reference to it as one of a class of facts of the war.

It is a secondary object of the recital to make evident, from narrations of actual experience, what is sometimes required for supplying the unavoidable deficiencies of government service in emergencies. Not to have sprung at once into a thorough practical knowledge of what the dread contingencies of war require, is no just cause of reproach to a peaceful

*The letters were all written by two officers of the Commission and six ladies serving with them. As the different writers are quoted from in succession, and the same occurrences are often described from more than one point of view, a capital letter at the head of a paragraph will indicate the change from one writer to another. The officers will be known by the letters A. and B.; the ladies, by the letters M. and N.

people like ourselves, who, meaning peace, sought only to "ensue it"; but not to thoroughly learn our duty under such an experience as we are passing through, would indeed bring shame upon our name.

It is no common nation's task that we have undertaken, and only craven souls will lose heart in finding that it cannot be light or short in the sacrifices which it demands of us. True and far-seeing lovers of their country, as they regard the sufferings of those uncomplaining men who fought for us in the Peninsula,—men who, though perhaps but green soldiers in the field, proved, one and all, heroes upon the bed of pain and in the hour of death, will be led to the reflection, "This is what it costs a republic to have nursed rebellion tenderly at its breast." We know that the barbarous spirit with which the chances of war first were dared in this gambling scheme of reckless ambition, will prolong it, when resistance to the law can no longer avail for anything but the gratification of the personal vindictive hate of the disappointed conspirators. And we know that if we do well the work the pecuniary cost of which we are throwing so heavily upon our posterity, this will be the last of such schemes. The more we feel its cost ourselves, the more resolute shall we be that, when done, this work shall have been done once for all. The more ready shall we be to meet whatever sacrifice it may yet require of us; the more ready to truly say, "Our loyalty is without conditions; success at this point or that, this year or next, we do not ask; we have elected our leaders, and we accept what they have the ability to give us. It is enough that in this nation, standing firmly upon its declaration of equal rights to all, no gleam of peace can ever be seen to fall upon a rebel in arms."

The deepest solicitude that all unnecessary suffering should be avoided in carrying on the war, is not in the least degree inconsistent with this sentiment, provided only it be guided and constrained by a true appreciation of the duties and the necessities of war. On the contrary, patriotism and humanity have one origin, and each strengthens the other in every heart. Whatever, then, leads the public to truly comprehend what the rebellion costs, and at the same time inculcates a right spirit of humane provision against the unnecessary suffering of war, must foster a sound and healthy public sentiment.

Such, it is hoped, may be the influence of this little volume, to the introduction of which only this further explanation will be required by the reader.

A sudden transfer of the scene of active war from the high banks of the Potomac to a low and swampy region, intersected with a net-work of rivers and creeks, early in the summer of 1862, required appliances for the proper care of the sick and wounded which did not appear to have been contemplated in the government arrangements. Seeing this, with the approval of the Medical Bureau, a proposal was made to the Quartermaster-General to allow the Sanitary Commission to take in hand some of the transport steamboats of his department, of which a large number were at that time lying idle, to fit them up and furnish them in all respects suitably for the reception and care of sick and wounded men, providing surgeons and other necessary attendance, without cost to government. After tedious delays and disappointments of various kinds,—one fine large boat having been assigned, partially furnished by the Commission, and then withdrawn,—an order was at length received, authorizing the Commission to take possession of any of the government transports, not in actual use, which might be at that time lying at Alexandria.

The only vessel then lying at Alexandria stanch enough for the ocean passage from Virginia to New York or Boston, proved to be the *Daniel Webster*, an old Pacific Coast steamer of small capacity. She had been recently used for transporting troops, and had been "stripped of everything movable but dirt,"—so that the labor of adapting her to the purpose in view was not a light one.

This vessel was assigned to the Commission on the 25th of April. Provisional engagements had previously been made, in New York and Philadelphia, with the persons afterwards employed as her hospital company. These were telegraphed for, the moment the order was received, and the refitting of the ship commenced,—at which point we turn to the narratives of those engaged in the work.

Chapter I.

(A.) Hospital Transport *Daniel Webster*, Cheeseman's Creek, April 30, 1862.

I received General Meigs's order under which this ship came into our hands on Friday. She was then at Alexandria, and could not be got over the shoals to Washington. It was not till near night that I was able to get a lighter, and this, after one trip, was taken off to carry reinforcements to McDowell at Fredericksburg. I succeeded before daylight of Saturday in getting a tug at work, and by the next morning, Sunday, had her hold full. At eleven o'clock got the hospital company on board, but the commissaries failed in their engagements, and at last I had to send off a foraging-party at Alexandria for beef. Finally at four o'clock, D., who had gone after E., and E., who had gone after beef, arrived simultaneously from different directions. With E. came the beef, and we at once got under way.

We had six medical students, twenty men nurses (volunteers all), four surgeons, four ladies, a dozen contrabands (field hands), three carpenters, and half a dozen miscellaneous passengers. There were, besides, five of us members of the Sanitary Commission and of the central staff, with one of the Philadelphia associates, eight military officers, ninety soldiers (convalescents, returning to their regiments), some quartermaster's mechanics, and a short ship's crew and officers. The ship has a house aft, with state-rooms for thirty, and an old-fashioned packet-saloon below, with state-rooms opening out of it; and all forward of the engine-rooms, a big steerage, or " 'tween decks," which had been fitted with shelves, some of them fifteen feet deep, in which the soldiers had been carried to the Peninsula, packed in layers.

I organized all our Commission people at sunset on Sunday, in two watches, sea-fashion; appointed watch-officers, and have worked since, night and day, refitting ship. We broke up all the transport arrangements,—they were in a filthy condition,—thoroughly scraped, washed, and scrubbed the whole ship from stem to stern, inside and out; white-washed the steerage; knocked away the bulkheads of the wings of the engine-room section, so as to get a thorough draft from stem to stern; then set to fitting and furnishing new bunks; started a new house on deck, forward; made and fitted an apothecary's shop; and when we arrived at Cheeseman's Creek were ready for patients.

(M.) It was a bright day, the river peaceful and shining. Just as we started, the little gunboat *Yankee* passed up, bringing, all on a string, five rebel craft which she had just taken in the Rappahannock. Late in the afternoon we passed the "stone fleet," eight boats, all ready to sink in the channel, in case the *Merrimack* should try to run up the Potomac. The rebels having taken up all the buoys, at dark we had to come to anchor.

Sunday, the first day, was gone. As for us, we had spent it, sitting on deck, sewing upon a hospital flag, fifteen by eight, and singing hymns to take the edge off of this secular occupation. Just after we had anchored, a chaplain was discovered among the soldiers; and in half an hour we got together for service, and an "unprepared" discourse upon charity, much like unprepared discourses in general. Quite another thing was the singing of the contrabands, who all came in and stood in a row so black, at the dark end of the cabin, that I could see neither eyes nor teeth. But they sung heartily, and everybody followed them.

(A.) *Cheeseman's Creek.*—I went ashore to report our arrival to the Medical Director. On our way up the harbor,—a shallow river-mouth, with low, pine-covered banks, in which there are now about four hundred steamboats and small transport craft,—I hailed the steamboat *Daniel Webster* No. 2, which carries the Regiment New York Volunteers, and let the Colonel know that his wife was among our nurses. This morning I received his acknowledgments in the form of a check for $1,000 for the Commission, accompanied by what was still better, a note of the most hearty and appreciative recognition of what the Commission had done for the relief of the soldiers.

Picking our way among all the craft, and keeping out of the way of the tugs and tenders which were flying about, we landed on a large meadow where were a number of wall-tents, one labelled "Office of Quartermaster's Department"; another, "Telegraph Office"; another, "Post-Office"; another, "Office of Land Transportation"; another, "Harbor-Master," &c., &c. One contained a number of prisoners, brought in the day before, and, of course, well-guarded. Ordnance and forage barges lay along the shore, with a few big guns, and piles of shot and shell, just landed. The ground was crowded;—orderlies holding horses; lounging, dirty soldiers; idlers and fatigue-parties at work in relays; sentries; Quartermaster's people, white and black; and a hundred army wagons loading with forage and biscuit-boxes from the barges. I went at once to Colonel Ingalls, at the Quartermaster's office. He was kind, prompt, decisive; horses were ordered for us, and we soon rode off through a swamp-forest, the air full of the roar of falling trees and the shouts of teamsters and working-parties of soldiers, the former trying to navigate their wagons, and the latter making corduroy roads for them.

The original country roads had all been used up; it was difficult even to ford across them, when we had occasion to do so, on horseback. The army wagons, each drawn by six mules, and with very light loads, were jerked about frightfully. We passed many wrecks, and some horses which had sunk and been smothered. Some wagons were loaded with gun-beds and heavy rope screens for embrasures; and we saw eight or ten mortars, each on a truck by itself, and drawn by from sixteen to twenty-four horses. At the first open ground we found cavalry exercising; then a cavalry camp, then a bit of wood, then rising dry ground, and our road ran through more camps. Then, coming in the midst of these camps, to the crest of a low swell, we opened suddenly a grand view of the valley of York River, a country something like the valley of the Raritan, at Eagleswood and opposite, but with less wood, more piny and more diversified, the river much broader, a mile and a half, perhaps, across. On the slope before us—nearly flat, with an inclination toward the river—was a space of several hundred acres, clear land, and a camp for some twenty to forty thousand men; shelter-tents, and all alive. It was a magnificent scene, the camp and all beyond, as we came upon it suddenly—right into it, at full gallop. The military "effect" was heightened now and then by a crashing report of artillery.

In the midst of the camp we came upon a long rack,—a pole on crotched sticks,—at which were fastened a score or more of horses. "We must stop here," said Dr. C. "They don't let you ride in." And that was all to show that we had reached Head-quarters.

It was an aristocratic quarter of the town, when you came to look at the clean tents and turf, but there were no flags or signs to distinguish it. We walked to the tent of the Medical Director, and just then there came another of those crashing reports. "They have been keeping that up all night," said the Doctor. "That isn't the enemy?" "Yes." "Is he so near?" "O yes! we are quite within range here."

The medical arrangements seem to be deplorably insufficient. The Commission is at this time actually distributing daily of hospital supplies much more than the government.*

(B.) *May 1st.* No patients on board yet; ship getting a final polish. Got up early and found the *Elizabeth* coming alongside for stores. The Commission has here at present, besides the *Daniel Webster*, one or two store-ships, and the *Wilson Small*, a boat of light draught, fitted up as a little hospital, to run up creeks and bring down sick and wounded to the transports. She is under the care of Dr. C., and has her little supply of hospital clothing, beds, food, &c., always ready for chance service. There is also a well-supplied storehouse ashore.

In sight are the abandoned rebel quarters at Shipping Point, now used as hospitals by one of our divisions; a number of log-huts finely built, but on low and filthy ground, surrounded by earthworks, which are rained on half the time and fiercely shone on the other half, and from which are exhaling deadly vapors all the time, a death place for scores of our men who are piled in there, covered with vermin, dying with their uniforms on and collars up,—dying of fever. . . . . .

I attended this afternoon to the systematic arrangement of the commissariat stores down aft, sent a telegram for more supplies to Baltimore, arranged for stowing the contrabands and putting bunks in the new deck-ward, and then put two ladies and a nice supply of oranges, tea, lemons, wine, &c., &c. on a small boat, and started them with —— to Ship Point Hospital, where four poor fellows died last night. Of course there is that vitally important medical etiquette to observe, here as elsewhere, and we must approach carefully, when we would not frustrate our own plans;—and so it is. "——, suppose you go ashore and ask whether it will be agreeable to have the ladies come over and visit the hospital,—just to walk

*See Appendix A.

through and talk with the men." So the ladies have gone "to talk with the men," with spirit-lamps, and farina, and lemons, and brandy, and clean clothes, and expect to have an improving conversation. After the party was off, sent orders to Fort Monroe for special supplies; received Dr. Tripler, who dined with us; furnished wine, tea, bread, to a surgeon who had been told that the Commission's flag was flying here, and had come seven miles across the swamps, and rowed out to us in a small boat to try for these things.

(M.) By dark the *Wilson Small* came alongside with our first patients, thirty-five in number, who were carefully lifted on board and swung through the hatches on their stretchers. In half an hour they had all been tea'd and coffeed and refreshed by the nurses, and shortly after were all undressed and put to bed clean and comfortable, and in a droll state of grateful wonder; the bad cases of fever furnished with sponges and cologne-water for bathing, and wine and water or brandy-toddy for drinking, and a man to watch them, and ward-masters up and down the wards, and a young doctor in the apothecary's shop, and to-day (May 3d) they are all better. . . . . .

Meantime additional supplies arrived from Washington, Baltimore, and Fortress Monroe, and a surgeon and nurses of our company were busy daily on shore at the Ship Point Hospital, dispensing stores, and doing what they could for the poor fellows there, who seemed to us in want of everything. . . . . .One hundred and ninety patients have now come on board; eighteen miles some of them say they have been brought in the ambulances (large statement of exhausted fellows jolted over corduroy roads). . . . . .We ladies arrange our days into three watches, and then a promiscuous one for any of us, as the night work may demand, after eight o'clock. Take Sunday, for instance.

It was ——'s and ——'s watch from seven to twelve. So they were up and had hot breakfast ready in our pantry, which is amidships between the forward and aft wards; ward-masters on the port and starboard sides for each ward, to watch the distribution of the food, and no promiscuous rushing about allowed; the number for coffee and the number for tea marked in the ward diet-books under the head of Breakfast, and the number for house-diet, or for beef-tea and toddy, &c., marked also; so that when the Hospital company learns to count straight,—an achievement of some difficulty, apparently,—there will be no opportunity for confusion. After breakfast we all assembled in the forward or sickest ward, and Dr. G. read the simple prayers for those at sea and for the sick. Our whole company and all the patients were together. It was good to have the service then and there. Our poor sick fellows lay all about us in their beds and listened quietly. As the prayer for the dying was finished, a soldier close by the doctor had ended his strife.

After twelve, our watch came on, and till four we gave out clean clothes, handkerchiefs, cologne, clothes to the nurses, and served the dinner, consulting the diet-books again. The house-diet, which was all distributed from our pantry, was nice thick soup and rice-pudding, and we made, over our spirit-lamps, the beef-tea and gruels for special cases. So with little cares came four o'clock, and with it clean hands and our own dinner; after which the other two ladies came on for the last watch, which included tea. Then there was beef-tea and punch to be made for use during the night; and so the day for us ended with our sitting in the pantry and talking over evils to be remedied, and should the soiled clothes be sewed up in canvas-bags and trailed behind the ship, or hung at the stern, or headed up in barrels and steam-washed when the ship got in? We crawled up into our bunks that night amid a tremendous firing of big guns, and woke up in the morning to the announcement that Yorktown was evacuated.

(M.) While we were lying anchored off Ship Point, down in the Gulf, New Orleans had surrendered quietly, and round the corner from us Fort Macon had been taken. What was it all to us, so long as the beef-tea was ready at the right moment?

Chapter II.

(A.) *May 5th.* On Sunday the *Ocean Queen*, coming up from Old Point, grounded about five miles off the harbor, and I went down and put a few beds and men on board to assume a footing. She had been brought to Old Point with the intention of using her to amuse the *Merrimack*, and had therefore been stripped of everything not necessary to the subsistence of the small crew.

(M.) On the way back, at eight in the evening, found that a great part of the army fleet, three hundred or more steamboats full of life, all before scattered for miles about the harbor, had been collected in close order and steam up. A number of heavy steamers swept past also, each with a tow a quarter of a mile long, making on the dark evening a long line of light and life. It was strange to see these floating cities melt away; the colored lights from the rigging going out one by one, and the bands and bugle-calls growing faint and far.

(A.) I had sent the *Webster* to sea, and with Mrs. —— and sister, B., and some two or three others, started in the *Small* to go to the telegraph and mail, and to bury the body of a patient who had died in the night. It was raining hard. When we reached the shore there was no post-office, no telegraph,—nothing of the military station left, except some wagons and transports. Our storehouse was a mile back. I left a portion of our party to move the goods from it on board the barge, and started in the *Small* for Yorktown, to which I presumed Head-quarters would have been moved. On getting out of the harbor, we saw that the *Queen* was underway. It turned out that she had been ordered to Yorktown by the Harbor-Master. As she was lying to, to sound the channel, we came up with her, and I went on board, after which—the *Small* going ahead to feel the way—we had a magnificent sail to Yorktown, the river so full of vessels that it was like getting up the Thames, only the lead was constantly going, "By the mark, five! A quarter less six!" and so on. Noble river! and a noble ship! Ahead, above all the fleet of three hundred transports, there were a dozen men-of-war. With our hospital flag at the fore, we slowly but boldly passed through the squadron, and came to anchor, the biggest ship of all, in the advance,—only one gunboat, as a picket-guard, being above us. I went ashore with the Captain and the young men, but could find no telegraph, and no officer of the general staff; and as many men had been killed and wounded by the torpedo-traps,—infernal machines set by the rebels,—we were not allowed to enter the fortified lines of Yorktown. So, picking up a hospital cot and stretcher left by the enemy, I took boat again to return to the ship, leaving the Captain and others ashore. As I pulled out through the vessels at the wharf, I saw to my surprise two small "stern-wheel" steamboats coming alongside the *Queen*, one on each side. Hastening on board, I found that these boats were loaded with sick men, whom an officer in charge was about to throw off upon the *Queen*. They were the sick of regiments which had been ordered suddenly forward last night, and which were at this very moment engaged in the battle of Williamsburg; we could hear the roar of artillery. They had been sent during the night by ambulances to the shore of Wormley's Creek, where a large number had been left, the officer assured me, lying on the ground in the rain, without food or attendance. His orders were to take them upon the "stern-wheelers," as many as both would carry, find the *Ocean Queen*, and put them upon her. I protested. The *Queen* at present was a mere hulk, without beds, bedding, or food even for her crew, and without a surgeon. It was obvious that the men were, many of them, very ill. Some were, in fact, in a dying state.

They were largely typhoid fever patients; and having been for twenty-four hours without nourishment, wet from exposure to the storm, and many of them racked by the motion of the ambulances over those frightful swamp corduroy roads (which I described the other day) into delirium, I was sure that many would die if they long failed to receive most careful medical treatment, with stimulants, nourishment, and warmth, no one of which could at that time be got for them on the *Queen*. The officer, however, insisted. I determined to go ashore to look for a surgeon, or if possible to find Colonel Ingalls, the transport quartermaster, a gentleman, and a most energetic and sagacious officer. I put the two ship's officers each at a gangway, with instructions to let no one come on board till I returned, and to use force, if necessary. I found a surgeon—a civilian—who was willing to help us, and pulled back, finding to my disgust, when I reached the ship, that the miserable first officer had given way, and every man who could walk of the patients had been taken on board. The glorious women had hunted out a barrel containing some Indian meal from some dark place where it had been lost sight of, in the depths of the ship, and were already ladling out hot gruel, which they had made of it; and the poor, pale, emaciated, shivering wretches were lying anywhere, on the cabin floors, crying with sobbing, trembling voices, "God bless you, Miss! God bless you!" as it was given to them from the ship's deck-buckets. I never saw such misery or such gratitude. My rebel stretcher came at once in play, and, after distributing forty dollars among the half-mutinous, superstitious beastly Portuguese crew and pantry servants, I got them at work bringing on the patients who were too feeble to be led on board. It was a slow and tedious process. By the blessing of God, before it was over, B., with Dr. Ware,—the two very best men I ever saw for such an emergency,—came with the *Elizabeth* from Cheeseman's Creek, and the Captain with the students from the shore. There were straw, bed-sacks and blankets, besides stimulants and medicines, on the *Elizabeth*, and the Captain's authority soon added all the ship's force to the working party on her, filling beds and hoisting out bales of blankets. B. went on shore, found a rebel cow at pasture, shot her, and brought off the beef, with another surgeon. By ten o'clock at night, every sick man was in a warm bed, and had received medical treatment; and beef-tea and milk-punch had been served to all who required it. But for three of them even the women could do nothing but pray, and close their eyes.

At half past ten, I went aboard the *Small*, intending to run to Fortress Monroe for additional supplies. It was stormy and thick, and I could not induce the Captain to go out till daylight. We reached Old Point about nine, A.M. I got breakfast in the hotel, and then to Head-quarters. While in the telegraph-room, a message was received, which was whispered between the operators; a minute afterwards a gun was fired, and the long roll beat; the infantry fell in on the parade, the artillery hurried to the ramparts and manned the heavy guns, and powder-carts were moving up the inclines. I asked, "What's all this?" "Telegram from Newports News that the *Merrimack* is coming out!" She did not come beyond Sewall's Point, however.

The boat from Baltimore brought six excellent New York surgeons, twenty-six nurses, and ten surgical dressers (medical students). I got them all on the *Small*, and having succeeded in obtaining the more important supplies in limited quantities, at noon left for Yorktown. On reaching here we found the "stern-wheelers" again alongside, and over three hundred patients on board; many very sick indeed, some delirious, some comatose, some fairly *in articulo*. The assistant surgeons, left behind at the abandoned camps, are too anxious to be rid of them, so as to move with their regiments, and have surgery of war. And as their orders authorize it, they hurry them off to us in this style, after a day's ride in army wagons, without springs, over such a country without roads as I described last week. They were horribly filthy, and there was no time to clean them, often not to undress them, as, sick and fainting, they were lifted on board.

About noon the next day I completed a hospital organization of such forces as I had, dividing the cabins and the upper steerage of the ship into five wards, for the bad cases, each ward having one surgeon, two ward-masters, and four nurses,—the two latter classes in watches; besides these, some assistant nurses and servants, convalescent soldiers, and contrabands. In these wards only the very sick—chiefly cases of typhoid fever—were taken. By cutting away bulkheads, and getting wind-sails rigged, they were fairly well ventilated. I had to offer $200 for the repair of damages before this could be secured, however. All the rest of the ship was the sixth ward, in which the hernias, rheumatisms, bronchitises, lame and worn-out men were placed, organized in squads of fifty each, with a squad-master to draw their rations of house-diet.

To get proper food for all, decently cooked and distributed, has given me more concern than anything else. The ship servants are brutes, and our supply of utensils was cruelly short. Fortunately the Captain is a good-hearted and resolute man, and the ladies—God knows what we should have done without them!—have contrived to make some chafing-dishes with which the kitchen is pieced out wonderfully. Just think of it for a moment. Here were one hundred miserably sick and dying men, forced upon us before we had been an hour on board; and tug after tug swarming round the great ship, before we had a nail out of a box, and when there were but ten pounds of Indian meal and two spoons to feed them with. No account could do justice to the faithful industry of the medical students and young men: how we all got through with it, I hardly know; but one idea is distinct,—that every man had a good place to sleep in, and something hot to eat daily, and that the sickest had every essential that could have been given them in their own homes. . . . .

B. was all this time driving everything to obtain supplies, while the sick kept coming faster than we could get anything ready for them. The last thing essential was more beef. B. at length got hold of a couple of draught cattle of Franklin's division, left behind in their advance by steamboats, and while these were being killed and dressed, we filled up to nine hundred patients.

To avoid having more pushed on board, I had the Captain heave short; so the moment that B.'s boat came, and the beef could be hoisted up, the steamer was underway, and before night, no doubt, was well out to sea.

I then went on board the *Small* to drop down quite ill for the time from want of sleep and from fatigue. A few hours' rest and a quiet dinner brought me all right, however, and at sunset I set out with B. to look after the sick ashore.

One of the strange effects, upon all concerned as workers on these hospital ships, in the heart of all misery and pain, and part of it, seems to have been the quieting of all excitement of feeling and of expression,— a sort of apparent stoicism granted for the occasion. A slight illustration of this quietness, which was characteristic of most of the hospital party, is given in the following passage from a letter of one of the ladies on the *Ocean Queen*:—

"It seems a strange thing that the sight of such misery, such death in life, should have been accepted by us all so quietly as it was. We were simply eyes and hands for those three days. Great, strong men were dying about us; in nearly every ward some one was going. Yesterday one of the students called me to go with him and say whether I had taken the name of a dead man in the forward cabin the day he came in. He was a strong, handsome fellow, raving mad when brought in, and lying now, the day after, with pink cheeks and peaceful look. I had tried to get his name, and once he seemed to understand, and screeched out at the top of his voice, 'John H. Miller,' but whether it was his own name or that of some friend he wanted, I don't know; we could not find out. All the record I had of him was from my diet-list: 'Miller,—forward cabin, port side, number 119. Beef-tea and punch.'

"Last night Dr. Ware came to me to know how much floor-room we had. The immense saloon of the aft cabin was filled with mattresses so thickly placed that there was hardly stepping-room between them, and as I swung my lantern along the rows of pale faces, it showed me another strong man dead. N. had been working hard over him, but it was useless. He opened his eyes when she called 'Henry' clearly in his ear, and gave her a chance to pour brandy down his throat; but all did no good; he died quietly while she was helping someone else, and my lantern showed him gone. We are changed by all this contact with terror, else how could I deliberately turn my lantern on his face, and say to the doctor behind him, 'Is that man dead?' and then stand coolly while he examined him, listened, and pronounced him 'dead.' I could not have quietly said a year ago, 'That will make one more bed, then, Doctor.' Sick men were waiting on deck in the cold, though, and every few feet of cabin floor were precious. So they took the dead man out, and put him to sleep in his coffin on deck. We had to climb over another soldier lying up there quiet as he, to get at the blankets to keep the living warm."

The business of feeding men by hundreds at short notice, in confined spaces, and with the aid of very limited cooking facilities, is one which can hardly be appreciated by those who have only heard, not seen, how it is accomplished. It takes good heads as well as good hearts, strong will as well as strong limbs, to avoid ruinous confusion. After a battle, when men are brought in so rapidly that they have to be piled in almost without reference to their being human beings, and everyone raving for drink first and then for nourishment, it requires strong nerves to be able to attend to them properly. Habit and system are the two great aids,—or rather system first of all, if possible; though system in such cases grows out of experience. Happily system has ruled in the work of the Sanitary Commission, and such success as has attended its operations is chiefly due to this, as every one must have observed who had an opportunity to witness the difference between its doings and those having the same end in view, but carried on without well-studied or sufficiently comprehensive plans.

But in these Atlantic Floating Hospitals the difficulties were very great. The desideratum is a practicable diet, simple yet nourishing, abundant and not injurious; always ready, yet varied enough to avoid the danger of satiety, which is ever threatening the sick man, whose chance of recovery may hang on his ability to eat his food with relish. In this arduous part of the Hospital Transport duty, the ladies were able to be especially useful; their sympathy and good judgment coming constantly in play, and the supply of fruits, jellies, and a variety of delicacies being generally so liberal as to afford full scope to their powers. But in dealing with hundreds and thousands of men, many of whom are not particularly in danger, but yet obliged to lie in beds for wounds to heal, it is necessary to provide on a scale so large as puts mere delicacies, or the ordinary resources of the sick-room, quite out of the question. It is utterly futile to attempt treating each one of four or five hundred patients as if we had him alone in a private family; and patients, as well as nurses and friends, must learn this after very little experience. But it is practicable here, as elsewhere, to accomplish much that is beneficial and comfortable by judicious system firmly carried out. To avoid collisions, and vain attempts to perform impossibilities, after a short experience, but careful study of what was really needed, rules were established which proved in practice nearly perfect in the matter of preventing delay and disappointment, while the result satisfied the patients in general quite as well as we can hope to satisfy sick men who have fitful appetites. As the suggestion may prove applicable to other cases, the established routine is given in full in the Appendix (B.).

Chapter III.

Just before the *Ocean Queen* left, a reinforcement of ladies and servants arrived from New York. A part of these were put on the *Queen*; temporary quarters were found for the remainder on the *Wilson Small.* Sick men were at this time being carted into Yorktown from the various abandoned camps in the vicinity, and the Sanitary party going on shore after the departure of the *Queen*, these were found lying in tiers in the muddy streets, while tents were being pitched and houses cleared for their accommodation. Several wagon-loads of hospital supplies were sent to them from the store-boats of the Commission; twenty-five dollars were given to the surgeon in charge, to be used to stimulate the exertions of his limited force of attendants, and for the purchase of odds and ends, and he was informed that, if more should be required, it would be provided by the Commission, and then the company started on their little boat for West Point, where a battle was reported in progress.

(M.) *West Point, May 9th.*—We arrived here early this morning. The whole field of battle is open like a map before us. A white flag flies from a small house just below us. We are along-side a transport on which an officer was yesterday wounded by a shell thrown from a battery which had been concealed behind this house, upon which the same flag was then flying. Another transport near us has a shot-hole through her smoke-stack. There are three or four thousand men along the shore, and more constantly arriving and disembarking by the pontoons, with artillery and horses. As I write, a blue column is moving off, the bayonets glistening far into the woods. We are sending off small stores, called for by the Commission's Inspectors ashore, who are visiting the extemporized hospitals, and are also supplying some of the gunboats' sick-bays with fruits and ice.

Just here a steamboat, loaded with sick and wounded, came along-side of us; a transport, made use of as a hospital on the occasion, but needing almost everything.

The more dangerously wounded upon this transport were transferred to the *Small*, and three ladies, with surgical dressers and servants, beef-tea, lemonade, ice, and stimulants, went to the assistance of the others, remaining with them till, after a transshipment at Yorktown, they were lodged in shore hospitals at Fortress Monroe.

(A.) The *Small* received the dangerous cases, several of amputation among them; the operations had been performed on the field. One died at midnight. I had great difficulty, at first, in our now very crowded little boat, restraining individual zeal within the requirements of order and tranquility; but I believe I succeeded, and as soon as the women began to experience the value of the discipline, they fell into it finely, and all behaved in the best manner possible. I put those on our boat in watches, rigidly excluding from that part of the boat where the wounded men were placed all who were not absolutely required on duty. The poor fellows were nearly all soon coaxed asleep, and the man who died passed away, and his body was removed without its being known to his nearest neighbor. We had on board Dr. Ware and two of the students, noble young fellows, zealous, orderly, and discreet.

I think all the men who have any chance for recovery look better this morning. One man (amputation of thigh) who seemed nearly gone when he came on board, staring wildly, and muttering unintelligibly, lifted his hand toward me as I came into the cabin this morning; and smiled when I bent over him. The nurse told me that he said to her on waking from a sound sleep, just at sunrise, "You have saved my life for my wife, good woman." There are several officers among them; one a hero, who led his company against a regiment, pushing it back, but losing one fifth of his men, and getting a shot through the lungs. There is Corporal C ——, too, who has lost his leg, and who says he bears no malice against the man who shot him, but he hopes some day to meet and punish the wretch who kicked him on his wounded leg, after he was laid helpless.

(M.) *May 11th.*—Three of our wounded men died during the night. Everything was done for them; they could not have had more care in their own homes. Our little boat is so crowded that the well sleep on the upper deck, all under cover being occupied by the wounded; and, the small outfit of china, etc. being needed for the sick, we take our meat and potatoes on slices of bread for plates, and make the top of a stove our domestic board.

As intelligence had come through telegraph from Washington that the *Ocean Queen* had been taken on her arrival at New York, against all remonstrance, for other purposes, the *S. R. Spaulding*, a large, seaworthy vessel, though lamentably inferior for a hospital to the magnificent *Ocean Queen*, was obtained in her place. She was fitted for carrying cavalry, with stalls for horses, and at this time filled with stable odor, and needed coal and water as well as complete interior reconstruction.

The *Daniel Webster*, arriving at Yorktown on her return from New York, could not get into the wharf-berth which had been secured for her near the hospital; a tug was consequently procured, which being run alternately with the *Small*, between sunset and twelve o'clock at night, two hundred and forty sick and wounded were taken off and put comfortably to bed. After this her hospital service was reorganized so as to transfer from her all the force that could possibly be spared, and to put on her any of the company whom it was necessary to part with. An estimate was made of the stores requisite for her home trip, and at daylight what she could spare was put on board the *Small*, and she steamed off on her second trip to New York, eighteen hours after she arrived. Everything is noted as going on admirably in the loading of the *Webster*, each man knowing his place, and not trying to do the duty of others. The discipline maintained by Dr. Grymes was most satisfactory, and the corps of ladies and nurses work as if they had been doing this thing wisely and well all their lives.*

At 9 A.M., the *Webster* started on her second trip, and there was time to look after the other vessels which were being fitted for the service. One company had been put at work on the *Elm City*, and another on the *Knickerbocker*, both these river boats having been handed over by the Quartermaster's Department to the Commission, to be fitted for hospital service. Stores had also been ordered to the *State of Maine*, a government hospital in need. All was found proceeding well with the limited force on the *Elm City*; but the *Knickerbocker*, where was she?

(M.) *Steamboat Knickerbocker*, *May 13th.*—If my letter smells of Yellow B, it has a right to, as my paper is the cover of the sugar-box. Since I last wrote we have been jerking about from boat to boat, fitting up one, and starting her off,

---

*Since the above was written, we have heard with deep regret of the death of Dr. Grymes. Wherever he served, his labors were singularly wise and efficient; with exceeding gentleness and quietness of manner he combined much energy of will, and to thorough skill was added a loving heart, and a rare devotedness of purpose.

then doing the same by another. We came on board this boat Saturday night. She had then about two hundred wounded men on board, taken from the Williamsburg fight, and bound for Fort Monroe, two of the ladies and assistants to look after the sick during the few hours' run, and others to get things on hand, and fit up the wards. We had fifty-six Commission beds made on the upper ward floor that night, and were ready to go on shore at Fort Monroe after the three and a half hours from Yorktown. Dr. C. came on board and had all the men carefully removed to the Hygeia Hospital, and we improved the opportunity to get some roses from the garden for our wounded men left on the *Small*, and to see Mr. Lincoln driving past to take possession of Norfolk. We lay at the fort all night, and were blown awake the next morning by the explosion of the *Merrimack*, when I found to my amazement that along-side of us lay the *Daniel Webster*, No. 2, Government hospital, with four or five of our Commission company on board, whom we had left at Yorktown. She ran, in passing, along-side our supply ships (all our boats of the Sanitary Commission are known by their flags,) just after we came away and begged for help. Mr. A. tossed on board everything necessary, including two ladies, two surgeons, and blankets, and started them off after us to the Fortress, with two hundred badly wounded men. They had been wholly uncared for till our people got on board. They did all they could for them in so short a time, washed them, gave them good suppers and breakfasts, and Drs. W. and W. dressed the worst wounds, watching them all night as tenderly as women could. This boat was all the next day unloading her sick; they were miserably wounded, and had to be lifted with great care. We on the *Knickerbocker* started up the river again, and anchored off Yorktown. . . . .We wanted a stove for our hospital kitchen on board, which has to be kept distinct from the kitchen of the ship's crew; so we went ashore with —— to seize upon anything we could find; poked about in all the rebel barracks, asked all the soldiers we met about it, and finally came upon the sutler's hut,—sutler of the *Enfans Perdus*, who was cooking something nice for the officers' mess over a stove with *four* places for pots! This was too much to stand, so under a written authority given to "Dr. Olmsted" by the Quartermaster of this department, we proceeded to rake out the sutler's fire and lift his pots off,—and he offered us his cart and mule to drag the stove to the boat, and would take no pay. So, through the wretched town, filled with the *debris* of huts and camp furniture, old blankets, dirty cast-off clothing, smashed gun-carriages, exploded guns, vermin and filth everywhere,—and along the sandy shore covered with cannon-balls, tossed into the river, and rolled back,—we followed the mule, a triumphant procession, waving our broken bits of stove-pipe and iron pot-covers. I left a polite message for the "Colonel perdu,"—which had to stand him in place of his lost dinner,—and I shall never understand what was the matter with that sutler, whose self-sacrifice secured our three hundred men their meals promptly.

The next morning the *Knickerbocker*, to the surprise of the Commission, was not to be found. They searched the fleet twice through for us, but in vain, and finally heard at the Quartermaster's office, that a requisition had been received at midnight for a boat to go at once to the advance of the army, on the Pamunkey River, and the *Knickerbocker* had been taken for it, the fact of her having been assigned to the Commission being entirely forgotten. The only mitigation of the anxieties of those who remained, for the ladies on board, was the assurance that the boat would soon return. Meantime, we, on board, sailed up the Pamunkey, getting a fine chance to perfect the hospital arrangements. We unpacked tins and clothing, filled a linen closet in each ward, had beds put in order for three hundred, got up our stove, set kitchen in order, filled store closets, and arranged a black-hole with a lock to it, where oranges grow, and brandy and wine are stored box upon box; and on reaching Franklin's head-quarters, the messenger transacted his business, we landed a file of soldiers and a surgeon of the division, who had shown us great kindness on the voyage, and were allowed to push off again unmolested. The army lay all along the shore, and General Franklin's head-quarters were in a large store house back from the river. We found on our return to Yorktown every one at work fitting up the *Spaulding.*

An order had been obtained from the Quartermaster for the planks and boards of some rebel platforms, with which to put up bunks, etc., and a gang of contrabands were set at the business. While this was going on, a visit was made to the surgeon in charge of the shore hospitals, with whom, after debate, it was agreed that the *Elm City* should be made ready by two o'clock to take on the sick who were waiting transport near the shore. The *State of Maine* was at the same time to be supplied and made ready to follow without delay. Going on board the *Small* again to carry out these arrangements, A. was met by a note from the Quartermaster enclosing a telegram from the Medical Director of the army at Williamsburg, demanding a boat provided with "*straw and water to be ready to take on two hundred sick and wounded within two hours at Queen's Creek.*" The despatch concluded, "This is of the utmost urgency. See the Sanitary Commission." The only boat in the fleet that had a fair supply of water on board was the *Elm City*, already assigned for other duty, and she had no stores of food. There was about one days' supply of provisions for two hundred men on the *Small*, and A. wrote at once to the surgeon in charge of the shore hospitals, that, to meet an order of the Medical Director, it had become necessary to change the arrangements just before made with him. He would have to withdraw the *Elm City*, but as supplies could be sent immediately to the *State of Maine*, she could be got ready before night to take her place. The *Small* was then put in motion, and first the *Elm City* was hailed in passing, with orders to "fire up and heave short, and be all ready to move in half an hour," thence to the *Alida*, which was sent with the supplies to the *State of Maine*, and then back past the *Elm City*, ordering her to follow, and so in good time up to the mouth of Queen's Creek, by the side of the *Kennebec*, loading with wounded Secession prisoners, brought out of the creek by light-draft stern-wheelers. The process of embarkation, witnessed at a point some distance up the creek, was rude, careless, and quite unnecessarily painful; the miserable wretches of rebels being made to climb a plank, set up at an angle of forty-five degrees, which they could only do by the aid of a rope thrown to them from the deck. Strange to say, they themselves made no complaint, but appeared to think that they were well treated. So much for habit. The only assistance the Commission could render was to make the pathway less slippery by nailing cleats closely together across the steep planks. To do this, nails were bought of an old man nearby, who at first asserted decidedly that not a nail could be found on his premises, until he was offered one dollar for twenty-five, when an abundant supply was discovered.

Notwithstanding the Medical Director's telegram, that the case was one of the "utmost urgency," no sick men were found at the place of embarkation on the creek, nor could any be heard of nearer than at Williamsburg. Proceeding thither, with great difficulty,—passing on the way directly through the field of the late battle,—A. inquired of the first man he met after entering the town, "Where is the hospital?" "The hospital, sir? Every house in the town is a hospital; you cannot go amiss for one." And this seemed to be literally true. Finding the Medical Director, he learned that he thought it important to relieve the hospitals by transportation as fast as he, in any way, could; but not supposing it possible that the telegraphic order could be literally complied with, he had taken no measures as yet to send the two hundred patients in question to the place appointed for embarkation. It was agreed, however, that a convoy of ambulances should be started at daylight, and A. returned to the mouth of Queen's Creek, and dispatched B. with the *Small* to Yorktown to bring up additional stores from the *Elm City*, upon which the half-completed work of filling bed-sacks and other preparations also continued through the night. With the first boatload of the wounded brought off in the morning, arose one of those conflicts of authority which so often embarrassed the Commission at this time in its work.

(A.) At the first step I was met by a Brigade Surgeon coming on board from the *Kennebec*, who went along giving orders over my head, changing my arrangements. As he persisted, and refused to compromise after I showed my written authority from the Medical Director, I told him that I should allow no sick to come on board until I was satisfied with the arrangements. He then declared that he should go to the Medical Director. "The very thing I want, and I will go with you. Meantime the sick, if any arrive, shall come on board, and Dr. Ware, here, will see to their disposition, if you please." He assented, and we then went to the landing and saw the lighter again loaded with sick, in the same manner as yesterday. When she was full, the surgeon said he should return upon her to the *Elm City*. "But I thought we were to go together to the Medical Director, sir!" "I have concluded not to do so, but have written to inform him that my authority is questioned." I deemed it best, after this, to go again to the Medical Director myself, and, after a tedious delay, got passage on a forage-wagon loaded with oats. What with the continuous atmosphere of thick yellow dust, and the jar of the heavy wagon over execrable roads, this was a hard ride.

I found the Medical Director, got a copy of an order which the Brigade Surgeon should have received yesterday, but which had failed of transmission to him, which failure justified officially his assertion of authority over *any* transport coming at that time to that anchorage.

Returned to the landing, and, the lighters having grounded, waited there, on the bank of the creek, with a hundred sick men, being devoured by mosquitoes and sandflies. On reaching the *Elm City*, found that, owing to the conflict of authority, and consequent imperfect system, as well as to the insufficient number of attendants, the sick were but slowly and with difficulty taken care of. Including the hundred coming off with me, the number on board was already over four hundred, or twice as many as the Medical Director had estimated, or I had had reason to calculate on in the supply of water, medicine, and stores.

After sunset I went again up the creek, and found eight men on the beach, left there sick, without a single attendant or friend within four miles, while, only the night before, two of our teamsters had been waylaid and murdered, as was supposed, by the farmers of the vicinity (guerilla fighting as they call it), in the edge of the neighboring woods. After taking them on board the small boat, I asked who had charge of the party, wishing to make sure that no stragglers were left. A man was pointed out, who, because he was stronger or more helpful than the rest, seemed to have been regarded by them as their leader, though he had no appointment. He was able to answer my inquiries satisfactorily, and then as he sat by my side, while I steered the boat, he told me about himself. His name was Corcoran. After the battle of Williamsburg he felt sick. There was an order to march, but his Captain said, "Good God! Corcoran, you are not fit to march. Go into the town and get into a hospital." He walked three miles carrying his knapsack, and when he came to a hospital the surgeon told him he must bring a note from his Captain, and refused to receive him. He went out, and, as he was now very ill, he crawled into something like a milk-wagon and fell asleep. He was awakened by a man who pulled him out by his feet, so that he fell heavily on the ground and was hurt. He begged the man—a Secessionist, he supposed—for some water, and he gave him some; and when he saw how sick he was, he said he would not have pulled him out only that he wanted to use his wagon. Corcoran then tried to walk away, but had not gone far when he fell, and probably fainted. By and by a negro man woke him up, and asked if he should not help him to a hospital. The negro man was very kind, but when they came to a hospital the doctor said he could not take him in, because he "hadn't a bit of a note." Corcoran said, "For God's sake, Doctor, do give me room to lie down here somewhere; its not much room I'll take anyhow, and I can't go about any longer!" It was then three days since he had tasted food. The doctor told him he could lie down, and he had not been up since till to-day.

I have repeated the whole of this story as I heard it, while we were floating slowly down the river, because the poor man who told it me died soon after we got on board, kindly attended in his last moments by our Sisters of Mercy. A letter to his mother was found in his pocket, and one of the ladies is writing to her.

This morning we returned to Yorktown, and took on the *Elm City* thirty more sick from a steamboat which had brought them from Cumberland on the Pamunkey.

At ten o'clock the *Elm City* left for Washington with 440 patients. . . . . After noon I went ashore, called on the surgeon in the charge of the hospitals and the Military Governor, made our arrangements for a trip up the river to collect scattered sick, and to tow our *Wilson Small* up to West Point for repairs. She has been knocked into and run against by all the big boats till she is completely disabled. Returning on board for this purpose, was met by an officer with a telegram, begging that a boat might be immediately dispatched to Bigelow's Landing, where an ambulance-train master had reported that "a hundred sick had been left on the ground in the rain, without attendance or food, to die." Bigelow's Landing being up a narrow, shoal, crooked creek, we ran about the harbor looking in vain for a boat of sufficiently light draught to send there. At length we determined to take our whole Sanitary fleet to the mouth of the creek, and, leaving the *Alida* and *Knickerbocker* outside, try to get up with the *Elizabeth*, for we had no single vessel, large or small, in itself, suitably provided.

We ran to the *Knickerbocker*, but before we could get her underway a steamboat, in charge of a military surgeon, came along-side, and a letter was handed me, begging that I would take care of one hundred and fifty sick men who had been taken on at West Point early in the morning, and who had had no nourishment during the day. It was sunset, stormy and cold. I at first hesitated, on account of the greater need of those at Bigelow's Landing, but the surgeon in charge having induced me to take a look into the cabin, I changed my mind. The little room was as full as it could be crammed of sick soldiers, sitting on the floor; there was not room to lie down. Only two or three were at full length; one of these was dying,—was dead the next time I looked in. It was frightfully dirty, and the air suffocating.

We immediately began taking them on board the *Knickerbocker*. . . . . . It is now midnight. B. and Dr. Ware started with a part of our company and the two supply-boats, five hours ago, for Queen's Creek, with the intention of getting them to the sick at Bigelow's Landing, if possible; if not, to go up in the yawl and canoe with supplies and firewood, and do whatever should be found possible for their relief. Two of the ladies went with them. The rest are giving beef-tea and brandy and water to the sick on the *Knickerbocker*, now numbering three hundred.

(M.) The floors of lower and upper decks are covered with beds. The men all have tremendous appetites, lazily sleeping and eating,—never miss a meal three times a day. If it were possible to have great eating houses and wayside places, where volunteers could break down and sleep and doze for ten days or so, the men forced upon us by the medical authorities here and sent North would be doing good work in their regiments,—a good bath, seven days' rest, and twenty-one good meals are all they need. ——is housekeeper on this boat, and great pails of tea and trays of bread and butter, and rice and sugar, go all around the decks for breakfast. Good thick soup and bread for dinner, and breakfast repeated, at tea-time. "Peter," with six long-shore Maryland oystermen (darkeys) runs the hospital kitchen, and has a daily struggle for the daily bread with the incorrigible fellows who shirk work, and for each meal protest against everything, and have three times a day to be brought round by highly colored blandishments. The sickest men, especially the one hundred and fifty last taken on, have plenty of beef-tea and cool drinks, made in the ladies' pantry, and all of them are now undressed and in clean, comfortable beds.

(A.) I am quite at a loss to know what I shall do to-morrow. Unless additional force arrives we certainly cannot meet another emergency. It will not be surprising if this letter is found somewhat incoherent, for I have fallen asleep several times while writing it, hoping all the time that B. might arrive. We have a cold northeast storm and thick weather, and I conclude that his expedition is unable to get down, and I may go to sleep for the night. I have just been through the vessel, and find nearly all the patients sleeping quietly, and with every indication of comfort.

May 16th. I fell so soundly asleep, that, fifteen minutes after I finished writing the above last night, it had to be several times repeated to me before I could understand where I was and what it all meant when the officer of the watch came to tell me that the supply boats were making fast to us, with over a hundred more sick. Anchoring the *Alida* at the mouth, B. had attempted to get up the creek with the *Elizabeth*, but, as I had feared, she went aground. Going on with the yawl, he found one of the steam-lighters at anchor with over a hundred sick and wounded men lying on the deck, who were soaked, not merely with rain, but from having been obliged to wade out to her in water knee-deep. He learned that, further up the creek, a few men, too badly wounded to stand, or too weak to wade off to the boat, had been left behind. No persuasion could induce the captain to return for them, but a threat to report him at head-quarters, at length made him fire up and go back. Eight were found just where I found eight on my night trip up the same creek a few nights before, some in a nearly dying condition. Having brought them off to the lighter, and served stimulants to them, she was run down the creek to the supply-boats, the freight-rooms of which had, in the mean time, been as well as possible arranged to accommodate the patients.

One of the ladies engaged in this night expedition of the *Elizabeth* gives the following account of it in a letter to a friend.

(N.) Not a moment is lost,—Mr. B. would not even let me go for a shawl,—and the tug is off. The *Elizabeth* is our store-tender or supply-boat: her main deck is piled from deck to deck with boxes. The first thing done is to pick out six cases of pillows, six of quilts, one of brandy, and one cask of bread. Then all the rest is lowered into the hold. Meantime I make for the kitchen, where I find a remarkable old aunty and a fire. I dive into her pots and pans, I wheedle her out of her green tea (the black having given out), and soon I have eight buckets full of tea, and pyramids of bread and butter. The cleared main-deck is spread with two layers of quilts, and rows of pillows a man's length apart. . . . . . The poor fellows are led or carried on board, and stowed side by side as close as can be. We feed them with spoonfuls of brandy and water; they are utterly broken down, wet through, some of them raving with fever. All are without food for one day, some for two days. After all are laid down, Miss G. and I give them their supper, and they sink down again. Anyone who looks over such a deck as that, and sees the suffering, despondent attitudes of the men, and their worn frames and faces, knows what war is better than the sight of wounds can teach it. We could only take ninety; more had to go in a small tug-boat which accompanied us. Mr. B. and the doctor went on board of her, to give sustenance to the men, and in the meantime the *Elizabeth* started on the homeward trip. So the care of her men came to me. Fortunately only a dozen or two were very ill, and none died. Still I felt anxious; six of them were out of their mind, one had tried to destroy himself three times that day, and was drenched through, having been dragged out of the water, into which he had thrown himself just before we reached him. When we reached the *Knickerbocker*, Dr. Ware came on board, and gave me some general directions, after which I got along very well; my only disaster had been that I gave morphine to a man who actually screamed with rheumatism and cramp. I supposed morphine would not hurt him, and it was a mercy to others to stop the noise, instead of which I made him perfectly crazy, and had the greatest trouble in soothing him. We did not move them that night, and the next morning, after getting them all washed, I went off guard, and Mrs. M. and Mrs. N. came on board with their breakfast from the *Knickerbocker*, where the one hundred and eighty men were stowed and cared for. Soon afterwards my men were transferred to her. She still lies along-side, and we take care of her. She is beautifully in order; everything right and orderly. It is a real pleasure to give the men their meals. The ward-masters are all appointed, and the orderlies know their duty. She will probably leave to-morrow. . . . . . As for the ladies, they are just what they should be, efficient, wise, active as cats, merry, lighthearted, throughbread, and without the fearful tone of self-devotedness about them that sad experience makes one expect in benevolent women. We all know in our hearts that it is thorough enjoyment to be down here; *it is life*, in short, and we wouldn't be anywhere else (in view of our enjoyment) for anything in the world. I hope people will continue to sustain this great work. Hundreds of lives are being saved by it. I have seen with my own eyes, in one week, fifty men who must have died anywhere but here, and many more who probably would have done so. I speak of lives saved only; the amount of suffering saved is incalculable. The commission keep up the work at great expense. It has six large vessels now running from here. Government furnishes these, and the bare rations of the men, (or is supposed to do so,) but the real expenses of supply fall on the Commission; in fact, *everything* that makes the power and excellence of the work is supplied by the Commission. If people ask what they shall send, say, "Money, *money*, stimulants, and articles of sick-food."

(A.) I went through the *Elizabeth* soon after she came along-side, and all who were awake were very ready to say they wanted for nothing. We concluded to let them remain where they were for the rest of the night. They had been on the creek shore from ten to fourteen hours, without a physician or a single attendant, a particle of food or a drop of drink, and this on a cold, foggy day, with rain and mist after nightfall. With half a dozen exceptions, they are marvelously well this morning, and profoundly grateful for the kindness which, I need not say, the ladies are extending to them. I am as yet unable to make up my mind what to do with them. The cold northeasterly storm continues.

May 17th. Our poor little *Wilson Small* since her first patching has been run into again and again, and for some days has been so broken up, that the poor little thing can't raise steam even. We have been towed about by our supply boats, and to-day shall quit her while she goes to Baltimore for repairs. We can't leave her without real regret, even to go temporarily on board the *Spaulding*, one of the finest vessels of her size that I ever saw. We go on slowly with our fittings, having but poor lumber and only four carpenters. We have had, however, a detail, ordered by the military governor, of the "Infant Purdys," as the boys call the *Enfans Perdus*, to fetch and carry, and shall have the *Spaulding* after next filling the *Daniel Webster* and the *Elm City*, both which should be here before to-morrow night. We sent off the *Knickerbocker* this morning at daylight to Washington, with two hundred and seventy sick and wounded. There are two ladies for each watch, and the value of their service in the minor superintendence is incalculable.

The twenty ladies who came from New York were really a great godsend, although at first, with no boat to assign them to, we did not know what to do with them. They have all worked like heroes night and day, and though the duty required of them is frequently of the most disagreeable and trying character, I have never seen one of them flinch for a moment. Yesterday, I chanced to observe, *apropos* to an excessively hard night's work, that all our hardships would be very satisfactory to recall by and by, when Miss M. said earnestly, "Recall! why, I never had half the present satisfaction in any week for my life before!" and there was a general murmur of concurrence. If you could see the difference between the men on our transports, and those on the vessels managed directly by government,—rude as the means at our command are, and although we do all we can to aid the latter,—you would better understand the incentive and the reward of exertion. . . . . The conduct of the patients is always fine;—patient, brave, patriotic. I am surprised and delighted by it. We have sent details of the ladies with every vessel, and have now remaining with us only four, besides the hired Crimean nurse, Mrs. ——.

Captain ——, whom I spoke of as mortally wounded, and whom we had kept in the cabin of the *Wilson Small* since our visit to West Point, we sent off this morning on the *Knickerbocker* feeling quite jolly and with a fair prospect of speedy recovery. I don't doubt he would have died but for good nursing and surgery, as he had exhausting internal hemorrhages.

We had two deaths on board last night,—one a fine fellow of sixteen, of pneumonia, in the lower deck ward, and a convalescent in the upper after ward. The latter came out of his room, saying he was faint, and wanted water, and, while the attendant turned for it, sprang over the guards into the water below. A boat was lowered and efforts made to find him, but he must have struck his head, and, being stunned, did not rise.

Chapter IV.

(A.) We are lying in the *Spaulding* just below a burnt railroad-bridge, on the Pamunkey River, and, as usual, in the middle of the fleet of forage boats. The shores are at once wooded and wonderful to the water's edge, the fulness of midsummer with the vivid and tender green of Southern spring. Up the banks, where the trees will let us look between them, lie great fields of wheat, tall and fresh, and taking the sunshine for miles. The river winds constantly,—returning upon itself every half-mile or so, and we seem sometimes lying in a little wooded lake without inlet or outlet. It is startling to find, so far from the sea, a river whose name we hardly knew two weeks ago, where our anchor drops in three fathoms of water and our great ship turns freely either way with the tide. Our smoke-stacks are almost swept by the hanging branches as we move, and great schooners are drawn up under the banks, tied to the trees; the *Spaulding* herself lies in the shade of an elm-tree which is a landmark for miles up and down. The army is in camp close at hand, resting, this Sunday, and eating its six pies to a man, and so getting ready for a move, which is planning in ———'s tent. Half a mile above us is the White House, naming the place,—a modern cottage, if ever white, now drabbed over, standing where the early home of Mrs. Washington stood. We went ashore this morning with General ——, and strolled about the grounds,—an unpretending, sweet little place, with old trees shading the cottage, a green lawn sloping to the river, and an old-time garden full of roses. The house has been emptied, but there are some pieces of quaint furniture, brass fire-dogs, &c., and just inside the door this notice is posted: "Northern soldiers who profess to reverence the name of Washington, forbear to desecrate the home of his early married life, the property of his wife, and now the home of his descendants"; signed, "A Granddaughter of Mrs. Washington"; confronted by Gen. McClellan's order of protection.

(M.) We were going up to head-quarters, but refrained, on consideration, and came back to the *Spaulding*, through army-wagons and pie-pedlers, and rewarded the three Generals who had come over to meet us with much-needed towels, handkerchiefs, and cologne. The river above us to the burnt railroad-bridge is crowded with steamboats and schooners. Four gunboats are our next-door neighbors. Beyond the bridge, round the corner, and out of sight, winds the Pamunkey, trees crowding down to the brink and dipping their feet in the water. The Harbor-master wanting the room in the evening, we dropped down the stream and anchored by a feathery elm-tree.

(A.) The next morning I saw the Medical Director at head-quarters. He seems to be in a worse boggle than ever as to the disposition of his sick. There are a great many still at Yorktown to be removed, but the work is now fairly systematized there, and the sick begin to collect *here* by hundreds, with a prospect of thousands, and no thought of system in disposing of them, as far as I can see. The Director has ordered us to take on men at once, but our bunks are not up, and I have promised him the *Daniel Webster* and *Elm City*, which should be here to-morrow, and can take six hundred. B. has gone down to bring up our boats from Yorktown, with all the stores that can be spared from our supply-ship. I shall try my best here to carry out the plan I have always wished to have pursued,—namely, the establishment of a large receiving hospital, from which those who really need to be sent away may be deliberately selected and transferred to proper vessels, properly equipped. During my visit this morning to the Medical Director's tent, four persons reported their arrival with sick, and were informed that there were no accommodations for them. Tents had been received, but there was no detail on hand to pitch them, and if they were pitched, there were no beds to put in them. Sickness was increasing rapidly, every case showing the influence of malaria. The Medical Director said, apparently with justice, that he had anticipated all this waste and confusion, and had made sample provision against it, but that almost none of his ordered supplies had reached him.

By night the *Daniel Webster* and *Elm City* had come up from Yorktown, and I went up with the first, securing with some difficulty a berth for her, and began taking on the sick at once, the Medical Director being present and superintending the embarkation. He seemed to have entirely lost sight of the plan about determined upon the day before, to establish the shore receiving hospital, and was only anxious to get the sick off his hands as rapidly as possible, being appalled by their accumulation and the entire absence of provision for them. Just at this time B. got back from Yorktown, bringing a cheering account of the hospitals there, and at the same time the arrival of large medical supplies and hospital furniture was reported, so that I had little difficulty in bringing about a return to the plan of yesterday.

The substance of the plan was this. The *Elm City*, able to accommodate four hundred patients, was to remain at White House as a receiving hospital; the *Spaulding* as a reserve transport in case of a battle; on the occurrence of a battle, the serious cases of sickness to be transferred to the *Spaulding*, and the *Elm City* used as receiving hospital for surgical cases; the *Knickerbocker* to remain as a surgical transport. If an engagement should occur at the close of the week, the *Spaulding* would take to sea three or four hundred sick, freeing the shore hospitals to that extent, making about six hundred with what the *Webster* would take; the *Webster* to return and take two hundred more the next week; the *Knickerbocker* to take two hundred and fifty every twenty-four hours to Fortress Monroe; thus relieving the shore hospitals to the extent of two thousand by the end of the next week, which would probably be all that was necessary. The *Webster* and *Spaulding*, being low between decks, crowded with berths, and deficient in ventilation, were not suited to the reception of sick and wounded for any other purpose than that of immediate transportation.

(A.) To relieve myself of further responsibility in case of another change of plan, I wrote a memorandum of what we expected to be able to do, and got the Director to sign his approval of it. He told me yesterday that he meant to have those who were to take ship carefully selected, and that he did not believe there were half a dozen who ought to go from here. I however saw being put on board the usual proportion of sick-in-quarters men, and told him. He attributed it to disregard of his orders by volunteer surgeons, a difficulty for which he declared that there was no remedy short of an act of Congress. I found Dr. ——, his chief executive officer, and got him to go to the sick camp, from which the men were being brought, when he discovered, as he afterwards told me, that the surgeon in charge had heard a report that the Sanitary Commission intended to have a receiving-ship here, and on his own responsibility (assuming that the *Webster* was to be used for this purpose) was sending men on board at random, and without reference to the gravity of their cases, his object being merely to get room. He also found that ambulances coming in from the advance had entered the train after it left the hospital, and the men thus brought to the shore were allowed to go on board with those brought from the hospital, as if assigned for sea transportation by the surgeon in charge. I begged him to go on board and send off such as he found of these interlopers, but he thought it impracticable; and finally, instead of the half-dozen proposed by the Medical Director yesterday, I found that he had passed two hundred and fifty on board. Meantime the tents before spoken of had been finally pitched on a large field near the White House. They were bare of everything but shelter for the sick flocking in from the different regiments. A thousand men will probably be in them before to-morrow night. All day long to-day the surgeons and young men of the Commission have been working over there, and we have sent over bed-sacks, straw, blankets, and supplies for several hundred. After much sanitary poking, pushing, and oiling, the tents are some of them floored, and five great pig-kettles are started boiling, and kept always full of food for the sick. The patients will, however, greatly overbalance the provision made for them. It is hard work to galvanize the proper authorities into action. The post hospital record certifies now to sixteen hundred. There are five surgeons and assistants, one steward, no apothecary, and no nurses, except those selected from among the patients. Two wells have been dug, but the water of neither has as yet been fit for using. Water is brought from the White House well, nearly a quarter of a mile distant, and until yesterday the whole supply was brought by hand. It is now wagoned in casks. We sent up three casks of ice from the *Webster's* stock, which was found of great value. The greater part of the men are not very ill, and, with nice nourishment, comfortable rest, and good nursing, would be got ready to join their regiments in a week or two; but this is just what they are not likely to have.

The weather is growing excessively hot, and the army is pushing forward in a malarious country in the face of the enemy. We have received a few wounded men from the skirmishes of yesterday. There is obviously great danger that we shall be altogether overwhelmed with sick and wounded in a few days. If the recommendation of my telegram of Sunday is adopted by the Surgeon-General, and a complete hospital for six thousand sent here from Washington, there will be reasonable provision for what is to be expected; otherwise it is dreadful to think of it. There is no doubt that we might take care of a few hundred on our boats,—probably save the lives of some of them; but considering what a week, or, for that matter, a day, may bring forth, I think it right to throw the authorities still on their resources as much as we can, and, if possible, force them to enlarge their shore accommodations. . . . . Nor, when ready, shall I be inclined to hasten the removal of the sick. I shall do my best to avoid taking any but serious cases. It is plain that the facilities so far offered in this respect have been abused, and that serious evils have come of it. Those responsible for the care of the sick here—I mean the military administrative as well as medical officers—have made the presence of the transports near them an excuse for neglecting all proper local provision, and evidently have the idea that, in hurrying patients on board vessels, they relieve themselves of responsibility.* I saw this danger from the first, and have (I wish the Surgeon-General and our friends to be sure of this) constantly done all that I could to counteract it, not only by verbal protest, but by a habit of action which I know that B. and other friends here, who have not had the duty of looking at the matter as comprehensively as I have, have not been able always to regard as justifiable. . . . . .

But this is not all. Of this hundred thousand men, I suppose not ten thousand were ever entirely without a mother's, a sister's, or a wife's domestic care before. They are wonderfully like school-boys. Then this is really the first experience of nearly all our officers (who are their schoolmasters and housekeepers) in active campaigning. They are learning to take care

*The reader must constantly remember that the Commission did not supply *vessels*, but merely furnished a few vessels already held by government with proper hospital arrangements, and that these were at the command of the medical authorities of the army, the Commission being responsible only for their internal administration.

of their men as a matter of self-interest. The men need to learn to make themselves content—of contented habit—away from home, to understand that this is in the bargain. It is obvious from the remarks we hear, that the rumor that sick men are to be sent home has a disturbing influence upon the education of the army in both these respects. . . . . .

The *Knickerbocker* has arrived while I have been writing; thus I have all the elements of my plan approved by the Medical Director on Monday. But the question still troubles me greatly, if they should have several hundred more patients on shore than they have tents or beds for, and among them all several hundreds seriously ill, such as would properly be sent North, shall I break up my reserve, and have no provision for the avalanche of suffering which a great battle before Richmond would send down upon us? I am afraid that I stand alone in my resistance to the demands of the present.*

As it has been publicly reported that the Commission removed forty thousand men from the Peninsula, it should be here stated that the total number of soldiers, sick and wounded, conveyed on the vessels in charge of the Commission, during the summer, was eight thousand. Except under positive orders, which it was not at liberty to disregard, the Commission took no patient on board its vessels until the opinion of a medical officer was had that his wound or illness was of such a character that he could not be fit for duty within thirty days. This was a standing order of the service, and was strictly enforced.

It is impossible to give in small compass an adequate idea of the difficulties of the duty which the Commission had taken upon itself; difficulties which, though seeming small in

*The wisdom of this resistance was satisfactorily established a few days later, as will be seen.

themselves, were terrible, because the lives of men frequently hung on their being overcome, and that instantly. To present a full picture, in true and living colors, we must be qualified to throw over the whole the atmosphere of sympathy and enthusiasm which animated every heart in presence of our suffering soldiers. On a fixed and recognized basis we can do almost anything; grooves are soon formed, in which affairs run smoothly. But to build with infinite toil on shifting sands; to be called upon to fill leaky cisterns and keep them full; to give our best strength to labors, the results of which often fade while we work,—these things require a great and good cause, and a certainty of being sustained.

(A.) All our vessels are, from the nature of engagement and intentions of those on board, in a constant state of pre-organization and disorganization. Our relations to the crews (seamen, firemen, &c.), upon whom we are dependent, differ in every vessel. Scarcely a day passes in which there is not a real mutiny among them, in which we have no right to interfere, but which it is necessary we should manage to control. We have scarcely any established rights, and are carrying on a very large business by the favor of a multitude of agents, whose favor in each case hangs upon a separate string. Every hour brings its own difficulty, which must be met by itself. . . . . . Except in the results accomplished, I need not say that the whole duty is exceedingly unpleasant, from the amount of dependence without rights, and of command without authority.

No two individuals have the same understanding of our duty or of our rights; no two expect the same thing of us; no two look in the same direction for the remedy of any abuse, or the supply of any organic deficiency to which attention is called. I must caution you again not to form theories of what we are to do, and expect us to do it. We are liable to occurrences every day which make a new disposition of all the forces necessary. In fact, new and previously unexpected arrangements are made daily, and these involve a continual modification of all plans. All that can be done is to be as fully prepared as possible for whatever can occur. . . . . . I must act a little blindly, sometimes,—at all events, cannot always give you my reasons readily for what I determine upon. Twice I have come up the river from hardly anything more than a crude notion that it would be prudent to be feeling that way, and would cost but little; and in each case it proved to be what —— calls "a *grand* good providence," leading to a complete change in our tactics, and to the saving of many lives. . . . . . The ladies are all, in every way, far beyond anything I could have been induced to expect of them. The dressers (two years medical students) are generally ready for whatever may be required, and work heroically. The male nurses are of all sorts. The convalescent soldiers have been the most satisfactory, because there was not among them the slightest taint of the prevailing sentiment of the volunteer nurses, that they were going upon an indiscriminate holiday scramble of Good-Samaritanism. There cannot be too much care in future that whoever comes here on any business comes, not to do such work as he thinks himself fit for, but such as he will be assigned to, and under such authority as will be assigned him. He or she must come as distinctly under an obligation of duty in this respect as if under pay, and must expect to submit to the same discipline. . . . . . But, in truth, I have had comparatively little trouble of this sort as yet, and in all respects am surprised at the good sense and working qualities of companies made up as ours has been.

As an illustration of the sudden changes of arrangement often found necessary at a moment's notice, a report is found, in which it is stated that on one occasion, after overcoming great difficulties in preparing the *Spaulding* for the conveyance of the sick,—having procured a party of thirty persons, including four surgeons and four ladies from New York, to go on board of her—on the 26th of May, while taking sick on board, an order was received immediately to remove all the Sanitary Commission's people and effects, and send her to Fortress Monroe to convey troops. The process of embarkation was at once arrested; but by permission of Colonel Ingalls, the post commander, the removal of those on board was delayed until an answer could be received to the following telegram, which was immediately dispatched to the Assistant Secretary of War, Mr. Tucker, then at Fortress Monroe.

(Telegram.) "The *Spaulding* was assigned to the Sanitary Commission after the *Ocean Queen* had been taken from them. The *Spaulding* was not well adapted to the duty, but was the only vessel then on York River which I would accept. There was no other, and there is none now here in which I would consent that a sick man should be sent outside. The hospitals at Washington and Alexandria are over full, and I suppose the sick must go outside if they are to be taken away. There is here no hospital but a few tents pitched by the sick themselves, in which robust men could not spend a night, crowded as they are, with impunity. There is not the first step taken to provide for the wounded in case a battle should occur. We have been two weeks trying, under great difficulties, to get the *Spaulding* tolerably fitted for the business; have a hospital corps of thirty, sent for her from New York; one hundred very sick men on board, one hundred more alongside; shall we go on, or quit?"

After waiting an hour, the Harbor-master's boat came past, hailing with "Mr. Tucker says, 'Go ahead,' sir!"—and the transshipment of the sick to the *Spaulding* from the *Elm City* was recommenced. The same night, as it appears from letters, just after dusk, the Harbor-master's boat appeared again, and Captain Sawtelle, the Master of Transportation, hailed with—

"I am ordered to have the *Elm City* and every other available vessel ready to leave here, with water and coal enough for eighteen hours' steaming, by break of day. You will oblige me very much if you will get the *Elm City* ready for me. How much coal has she on board?"

"Not half enough for eighteen hours' steaming!"

"That is bad. I have to coal half a dozen others tonight; there'll not be time for all."

"Very well, sir; then we'll manage it, by clubbing that which is on the *Knickerbocker* and the *Elizabeth*."

"If you can do that I shall be very glad, for the order is urgent."

(B.) We had just got through with a very long and hard day's work loading the *Spaulding* and were sitting at supper when this order came; but there was no help for it, so "All hands!" it was again for a hard night's work.

All the hospital fittings and furnishings of the *Elm City*, including the bedding, commissary and small stores, medical stores, and what not, required for the hospital treatment of four hundred and fifty sick men and the maintenance of their attendants, had to be unshipped, packed, and conveyed to the store-boats, and ninety sick men, some of them very sick indeed,—two died during the night,—to be transferred and put to bed again on the *Spaulding* and *Knickerbocker*. It was a very dark night, and most of those who were engaged in this work were men of sedentary occupations,—students and clerks,—and women accustomed to a quiet and refined domestic life, and, as I said, all had just gone through with an extraordinarily fatiguing day's work. Some few broke down before morning. At the same time twenty tons of coal were to be got on board the *Elm City* from the *Elizabeth* and the *Knickerbocker*, and wheeled to her deck-bunkers. Then quarters had to be found for her whole hospital company, as well as provisions, on the other boats of the fleet, and to accommodate this necessity a general reorganization was found to be necessary. This was our Sunday's night-work after our Sunday's day-work. It was all done, everybody in place, and, except those required to watch the sick, asleep by four o'clock, and the *Spaulding* (with 350 sick in bed) and the *Elm City* (stripped for battle) both reported ready to sail with the morning tide.

One day later, B. writes:—

"Here we are at work again upon the *Elm City*. Sunday, we spent all night in stripping her, and now we have a day and night's work at least before us in handling over again the very same articles, refitting her for hospital service. It is an exercise of patience, but it must be done without delay. After we had got her all ready for transporting troops, a change in the plans of government occurred, and on application she was again assigned to the Commission."

(M.) The *Spaulding* is bunked in every hole and corner, and is a most inconvenient ship for carrying sick men, everything above decks running to first-classing, and everything below to steerage. The last hundred patients were put on board, to relieve the over-crowded shore hospital, late last night. Though these night scenes on the hospital ships are part of our daily living, a fresh eye would find them dramatic. We are awakened in the dead of night by a sharp steam-whistle, and soon after feel ourselves clawed by the little tugs on either side our big ship,—and at once the process of taking on hundreds of men, many of them crazed with fever, begins. There's the bringing of the stretchers up the side ladder between the two boats, the stopping at the head of it, where the names and home addresses of all who can speak are written down, and their knapsacks and little treasures numbered and stacked;—then the placing of the stretchers on the platform, the rows of anxious faces above and below decks, the lantern held over the hold, the word given to "Lower!" the slow-moving ropes and pulleys, the arrival at the bottom, the turning down of the anxious faces, the lifting out of the sick man, and the lifting him into his bed;—and then the sudden change from cold, hunger, and friendlessness, to positive comfort and satisfaction, winding up with his invariable verdict,—if he can speak,—"This is just like home!"

"Jimmy," eleven years old, one of the strange little city boys who are always drifting about, ran away from home last summer, after a drum, finally turning up on our stern-wheeler as char-boy, where he recognized a friend among the sick men, and devoted himself to him in the prettiest way. His runaway fever over, he longed for his mother; so we tucked him into the *Spaulding* and sent him home. The astonishing lack of common sense among men strikes us very forcibly. . . . . . Those who came down here have hearts, plenty of them, but not more than a head to four, and so they run round the wards, wondering where the best tea is, and the ice water, which they are probably looking at, at the time, and ask questions about everything under the sun.

(B.) The *Spaulding*, being all in order, with her sick men, corps of nine surgeons, ladies, and nurses, was started off, and the reserve force went on board the *Knickerbocker*.

(A.) I have just bought what is left of a small cargo of ice, probably sixty tons, at twelve dollars, sent here on speculation for sale to sutlers. We are now fairly well supplied at all points, I think.

(A.) We began taking sick on the *Elm City* this afternoon. I telegraphed you about the crowded state of the post hospital. We had fed this morning sixty men who had been turned away from it on the ground that there was no room. I wrote to the surgeon in charge about this, and B. called on him with my note. He merely said that he thought there could not have been *as many* as sixty turned away! These sixty men we heard of as lying upon the railroad, without food, and with no one to look after them. So some of the ladies got at once into the stern-wheeler *Wissahickon*, which is the Commission's carriage, and with provisions, basins, towels, soap, blankets, etc., went up to the railroad-bridge, cooking tea and spreading bread as they went. After twenty minutes' steaming, the men were found, put on freight-cars, and pushed down to the landing, fed, washed, and taken on the tug to the *Elm City*. Dr. Ware, in his hard-working on shore, had found fifteen other sick men, without food, and miserable; there being "no room" for them in the tent hospital. He had studied the neighborhood extensively for shanties, found one, and put his men into it. The floor of the one room up-stairs was six inches deep in beans, and made a good bed for them, and in the morning the same party ran up on the tug, cooking breakfast for them as they ran, scrambling eggs in a wash-basin over a spirit-lamp.

(A.) The army struck its tents one night last week, and silently stole away up the river. Bottom Bridge is ours, and no enemy met; the railroad is repaired at White House, and trains will be running tomorrow; barges, loaded with rolling stock and cannon, have been passing us on the river all day.

The sick brought on board the *Elm City* this afternoon had been lying in a puddle, which nearly covered them. The water stood several inches deep in some of the tents. These men were selected by Dr. Ware, as the worst cases out of sixteen hundred in the shore hospital. (Several died before they reached the mouth of the river.) Dr. Ware himself laid hold to put up tents to protect men before the storm, and said that he saw half a dozen tents yet remaining, not put up at nightfall, though men were constantly arriving, and were left out in the ambulances.

If an engagement occurs this side of Richmond, my opinion is that we shall have all the horrors of Pittsburgh Landing in an aggravated form. I have tried in vain to awaken some of the Head-quarters officers to a sense of the danger; but while they admit all I say, they regard it as a part of war, and say, "After all, there never was a war in which the sick were as well taken care of. England does no better by her wounded; true, they will suffer a good deal for a time, but that is inevitable in war," &c.

What ought to be done? The Surgeon-General cannot at once do our sea-transport business as well as we. By recruiting deficiencies at each trip, we can for the present continue to employ the *Webster* and the *Spaulding* for this purpose advantageously. We can maintain the distribution of supplies. We want also a depot at this end for our sea-transports. For the rest, the Surgeon-General can at once have it done a great deal better than we, if he can place two steamboats under the Medical Director's orders, in addition to the *Com-*

modore and *Vanderbilt*, equip them, or take them equipped from us; put one good authoritative surgeon on board each, with two to four assistant surgeons, and six to ten dressers and stewards, and twenty to thirty privates for nurses, and require certain rules, to secure decent provision for the sick, to be maintained on them.

It is ludicrous to see the enthusiasm of some of the surgeons at the outset about details; the cleansing of patients, numbering, records of disease, *pure* water, &c., and their entire forgetfulness and inaptness to provide for more essential matters,—food, buckets, cups, vessels of any sort, and water of any sort. Doctors, nurses, and philosophers are much easier to be had, it seems, than men who would be able to keep an oyster-cellar or a barber-shop with credit.

Dr. T. says that he is pestered by volunteer surgeons, who leave their business at home to have a short holiday professional excursion, and who always expect to be put in the "imminent deadly breach" at once. He has not tents, horses, forage, nor table-room for them. Don't let any more surgeons come here, if you can help it. We try to treat them civilly, but all, ashore and afloat, feel anything but civilly to a man when he graciously proposes to be entertained and sent to the front as an honored guest, because, you understand, he is not one of your "physicians," but a "surgeon," and not all unwilling to take an interesting gunshot case in hand, though everybody else declines it! If there is anything the regimental surgeons hate, it is to let these magnanimous surgical pretenders (it is of the pretenders I speak) get hold of their pet cases. For this reason I hope ——, who has a name, will assume the responsibility of our surgical hospital.

Chapter V.

(A.) *May 31st.*—Sick men arriving Friday night by the railroad could not be provided for in the crowded field-hospital ashore, which still remained of but one fifth the capacity in tent-room which I urged it should be made three weeks ago. To make more room, on Saturday morning, 31st, we were ordered to take off four hundred upon the *Elm City.* They were sent to her by smaller steamboats, and the last load, which brought the number up to four hundred and fifty, arrived so late Saturday night that she could not leave till daylight Sunday morning. The orders were to deliver the men at Yorktown and return immediately. I urged Dr. ——, who was the surgeon in charge, and the captain and engineer to do their best, and telegraphed to have every preparation made at Yorktown.

June 1st.—We had sent out two parties to look for straggling sick, and visit the hospitals in the rear of the left wing. One of these returned at noon, having been by Cumberland to New Kent Court-House. From Dr. ——, who was in charge of the other, I received a dispatch about sunset, stating that his party were assisting the surgeons in a field-hospital, to which wounded were crowding from a battle then in progress. Soon after midnight this party arrived on board, having come from the front with a train of wounded, and we then had our first authentic information of the fierce battle in which our whole left wing had been engaged.

On that Sabbath day, after the departure of the *Elm City*, the wounded of the battle of Fair Oaks began to arrive in large numbers by railroad. After energetic remonstrances, with the responsible medical officer, on the part of the Commission, and a vain struggle to secure an adherence to some plan by which care and method in their shipment could be expected, a frightful scene of confusion and misery ensued at the landing, in the midst of which three government boats and two of those assigned to the Commission were loaded with wounded. We omit the painful particulars, because they could not be given without casting the gravest censure where censure would now be useless.* To understand the extracts which follow, it is only necessary to know, that so well were things managed on the *Elm City* (which, it will be remembered, left, loaded with sick, in the morning), that she had proceeded to Yorktown, discharged her sick, and returned with beds made, reporting ready to receive wounded at White House before sunset the same day.

(M.) The Commission boats were all here, and ready to remove the wounded of the battle of the 1st and 2d of June. They filled and left with their accustomed order and promptitude. After that, other boats, detailed by government for hospital service, were brought up. These boats were not in

*Some idea of the causes of the confusion at White House at this time may be formed from a communication addressed by the representative of the Commission to the Medical Director, of which a copy is given in the Appendix (C.). Together with a memorandum of arrangements suggested subsequently, to provide against its recurrence. The officer who seems to have been most palpably at fault at White House has since been publicly disgraced for a similar offense.

the control of the Commission. There was no one specially appointed to take charge of them, no one to receive the wounded at the station, no one to ship them properly, no one to see that the boats were supplied with proper stores. Of course the Commission came forward to do all it could at a moment's notice, but it had no power; only the right of charity. It could neither control nor check the fearful confusion that ensued, as train after train came in, and the wounded were brought and thrust upon the various boats. But it did nobly what it could. Night and day its members worked, not, you must remember, in its own well-organized service, but in the hard duty of making the best of a bad case. Not the smallest preparation was found, in at least three of the boats, for the common food of the men. As for sick-food, stimulants, drinks, &c., such things scarcely exist in the medical mind of the army, and there was not even a pail or a cup to distribute food, had there been any.

(N.) *June 5th.* . . . . We had been helping the ladies on the *Elm City* all night, had returned to our quarters, and just washed and dressed, when Captain —— came on board, to say that several hundred wounded men were lying at the landing,—that the *Daniel Webster* No. 2 had been filled, and the surplus was being sent on board the *Vanderbilt,*—that the confusion was terrible; there were no stores on board either vessel. Of course the best in our power had to be done. Our supply-boat *Elizabeth* came up. We begged Mr. —— not to refrain from sending us because we had been up all night; he said that he wouldn't send us, but if, in view of so much misery, we chose to offer our services to the United States surgeon in charge, he thought it would be merciful. We went on board, and such a scene as we entered and lived in for two days I trust never to see again. Men in every condition of horror, shattered and shrieking, were being brought in on stretchers, borne by contrabands, who dumped them anywhere, banged the stretchers against pillars and posts, and walked over the men without compassion. There was no one to direct what ward or what beds they were to go into. The men had mostly been without food since Saturday, but there was nothing on board for them, and the cook was only engaged to cook for the ship, and not for the hospital.

The first thing *wounded* men want is lemonade and ice (with the sick, stimulants are the first thing); after that, we give them tea and bread. Imagine a boat like the *Bay State*, filled on every deck, every berth,—and every square inch of room covered with wounded men,—even the stairs and gangways and guards filled with those who are less badly wounded,—and then imagine fifty well men, on every kind of errand, hurried and impatient, rushing to and fro over them, every touch bringing agony to the poor fellows,—while stretcher after stretcher still comes along, hoping to find any empty place; and then imagine what it was to keep calm ourselves, and make sure that each man on our own boat, the *Elm City*, and then on this, was properly refreshed and fed. We *got through* about one o'clock at night, Mrs. —— and Miss —— having come off other duty, and reinforced us. We were sitting for a few moments resting and talking it over, and bitterly asking why a government, so lavish and so perfect in its other departments, should leave its wounded almost literally to take care of themselves, when a message came that one hundred and fifty men were just arriving by the cars. It was raining in torrents, and both boats were full. We went on shore again; the same scene repeated. The *Kennebec* was brought up, and the one hundred and fifty men carried across the *Daniel Webster* No. 2 to her, with the exception of some fearfully wounded ones who could not be touched in the darkness and rain, and were, therefore, left in the cars. We gave refreshments to all; a detail of young men from the *Spaulding* coming up in time to assist, and the officers of the *Sebago* (gunboat), who had seen how hard pressed we were in the afternoon, volunteering for the night-watch. Add to this sundry members of Congress, who, if they talked much, at least worked well. We went to bed at daylight with *breakfast* on our minds. At half past six we were all on board the *Webster*

No. 2, and the breakfast of six hundred men was got through with before our own.

(A lady on the *Knickerbocker.*) *Sunday.*—"Three hundred wounded to come on board!" I wish you could see the three hundred white beds, with a clean shirt and drawers laid ready for each man. . . . . . They began to bring them in about noon. Many of them were shockingly hurt; but the men were proud of their wounds, and one of them, an artist, private of a New York regiment, was thankful that he had only lost a leg,—"so glad it wasn't his arm!" We went directly at work washing them, doing what we could, too, at dressing wounds which had been hastily bandaged on the battle-field thirty-six hours before. Men very patient and grateful always.

(A.) *Sunday Night.*—The *Knickerbocker* had, by estimate, three hundred and fifty on board. The night being fine, many were disposed of on the outer decks, and before I left, at eleven o'clock, nearly all had been washed, dressed, and put to bed decently, and were as comfortable as circumstances would admit of our making them. All had received needed nourishment, and such surgical and medical attention as was immediately demanded. Leaving the *Knickerbocker* in this satisfactory condition, I came back in a small boat, at midnight, to the landing, where I found that the *Elm City* already had five hundred wounded on board. I ordered her to run down and anchor near the *Knickerbocker.* There had been a special order in her case from the Medical Director to go to Washington. (I judge that this was given under the misapprehension that she had failed to go to Yorktown, and had her sick still on board.) She was unable to go at once for want of coal, which could not be furnished her till the evening of the next day (Monday). This finished the Commission's boats for the present. The *State of Maine* had been ordered to the landing by the Harbor-master, and the wounded remaining on shore, excluded from the *Elm City*, were flocking on board of her. Our ladies on the *Elm City* sent them some food, and we put on board from our supply-boat bedding and various stores, of which there was evident need, without waiting to be asked, and without finding anyone to receive them, the surgeons being fully engrossed in performing operations of pressing necessity.

The battle had been renewed in the morning of this day (Sunday), and we had sent a relief party, composed of medical students and male nurses, with supplies of stimulants, lint, etc., to the battle-field hospitals. A portion of this party returned about midnight, with another large train of wounded. All our force that could possibly be withdrawn from duty on the boats was immediately employed in distributing drink, and in carrying the wounded from the railroad to the boat. Some men died on the cars. I made another visit to the *Knickerbocker* in the morning, and on my return (Monday), found that a train had just arrived, and the wounded men were walking in a throng across the scow to the *Webster* No. 2, Government Hospital, the only boat remaining at the landing. I knew that she was not prepared for them, and sent for Dr. S., the representative of the Medical Director. Dr. S. could not be found. I asked for the medical officer in charge of the *Webster* No. 2. The Captain said there was none, and that he had no orders except to bring his boat to the landing. I inquired for the surgeon in charge of the railroad train, but could find none. There was no one in charge of the wounded. Meantime they were taken out of the cars, and assisted towards the landing by volunteer by-standers, until the gang-planks of the boat, the landing-scow, and the adjoining river-banks were crowded. I finally concluded that Dr. S. must have intended them to go on board the *Webster* No. 2. I could find no one in the crowd who professed to have received his orders, but, as many were nearly fainting in the sun, I advised the Captain to let them come on board. He did so, and they hobbled on, till the boat was crowded in all parts. The *Small* was outside the *Webster* No. 2, and our ladies administered as far as possible to their relief. Going on shore, I found still a great number, including the worst cases, lying on litters, gasping in the fervid sun. I do not describe such a scene. The worst cases I had brought upon the *Small*. Two died on the forward deck, under the shade of the awning, within half an hour. One was senseless when brought on; the other revived for a moment, while Mrs. G. bathed his head with ice-water, just long enough to whisper the address of his father, and to smile gratefully, then passed away, holding her hand.

. . . . . At the time of which I am now writing (Monday afternoon), wounded men were arriving by every train, entirely unattended, or with at most a detail of two soldiers, two hundred or more of them in a train. They were packed as closely as they could be stowed in the common freight-cars, without beds, without straw, at most with a wisp of hay under their heads. Many of the lighter cases came on the roof of the cars. They arrived, dead and living together, in the same close box, many with awful wounds festering and swarming with maggots. Recollect it was midsummer in Virginia, clear and calm. The stench was such as to produce vomiting with some of our strong men, habituated to the duty of attending the sick. How close they were packed, you may infer from a fact reported by my messenger to Dr. Tripler, who, on his return from Head-quarters, was present at the loading of a car. A surgeon was told that it was not possible to get another man upon the floor of the car. "Then," said he, "these three men must be laid in *across the others*, for they have got to be cleared out from here by this train!" This outrage was avoided, however.

Need I tell you that the women were always ready to press into these places of horror, going to them in torrents of rain, groping their way by dim lantern light, at all hours of night, carrying spirits and ice-water; calling back to life those in despair from utter exhaustion, or again and again catching for mother or wife the last faint whispers of the dying?

One Dr.—— was at this time the only man on the ground who claimed to act as a medical officer of the United States.

He was without instructions and without authority, and, though miraculously active, could do nothing toward bringing about the one thing wanted, orderly responsibility, and while he was there, ——, who might otherwise have done something, would not interfere. Dr. Ware, of our party, was at one time the only other medical man on the ground. The *Spaulding*, Dr. —— in charge, arrived Monday night, but not in a condition to be made directly useful, being laden with government stores, which could not at once be removed by the quarter-master. Her physicians and students, however, could never have been more welcome. I put one half her eager company at once at work on the *Webster No.* 2. Captain Sawtelle, at my request, pitched a hospital tent for the ladies at the river-bank by the railroad, behind which a common camp-kitchen was established. To this tent quantities of stores have now been conveyed, and soup and tea in camp-kettles are kept constantly hot there. Before this arrangement was complete, and until other stores arrived, we were for a time very hard put to it to find food of any kind to meet the extraordinary demand upon us. Just as everything was about giving out, B. found a sutler, who told him that he had five hundred loaves of bread on board of a boat which had just arrived at Cumberland, but he had no way of getting it immediately up. A conditional bargain was immediately struck, and the *Elizabeth* hastened off to Cumberland to bring up the bread. When it arrived, to our horror, it proved to be so mouldy it could not be used. B., almost crying with disappointment, started again to make a search through the exhausted sutlers' stores of the post. While doing so, he came upon a heap of boxes and barrels unopened and "unaccounted for." "What's all this?" "Sutlers' goods." "Who owns them?" "I do. I am the sutler of the——New York, up to the front. I want to get them up there, but I can't get transportation." "What's in here?" said B. in great excitement. "Mack'rel in them barrels." "What's in the boxes?" "That's wine biscuit. There's two barrels of molasses and a barrel of vinegar. I've got forty barrels of soft tack, too." "Where's that?" "That's one of 'em"; and B., hardly waiting for leave, seized a musket, and jammed a head off. It was aerated bread, and not a speck of mould upon it! He bought the sutler's whole stock on the spot, and in half an hour the ladies were dealing out bread spread with molasses, and iced vinegar and water. . . . .

The trains with wounded and sick arrive at all hours of the night; the last one before daylight, generally getting in between twelve and one. As soon as the whistle is heard, Dr. Ware is on hand (he has all the hard work of this kind to do), and the ladies are ready in their tent; blazing trench-fires, and kettles all of a row, bright lights and savory supplies, piles of fresh bread and pots of coffee,—the tent door opened wide,—the road leading to it from the cars dotted all along the side with little fires or lighted candles. Then, the first procession of slightly wounded, who stop at the tent-door on their way to the boat, and get cups of hot coffee with as much milk (condensed) as they want, followed by the slow-moving line of bearers and stretchers, halted by our Zouave, while the poor fellows on them have brandy, or wine, or iced lemonade given them. It makes but a minute's delay to pour something down their throats, and put oranges in their hands, and saves them from exhaustion and thirst before, in the confusion which reigns on most of the crowded government transports, food can be served them. When the worst cases have been sent on board, those which are to go to the shore hospital the next day are put into the twenty Sibley tents, pitched for the Commission, along the railroad, and our detail of five men start, each with his own pail of hot coffee or hot milk, and crackers and soft bread, with lemonade and ice-water, and feed them from tent to tent, a hundred men every night; sometimes one hundred and fifty are thus taken care of, for whom no provision has been made by government. Dr. Ware sees them all, and knows that they have blankets attendants, stimulants, &c. for the night. When the morning comes, ambulances are generally sent for them from the shore hospital, but occasionally they are left on the Commission's hands for three days at a time. They would fare badly but for the sleepless devotion of Dr. Ware, who, night after night, works among them, often not leaving them till two or three o'clock in the morning. The ladies from the *Webster*, and other Commission boats, visit the shore hospital between their voyages, and carry to the sick properly prepared soups and gruels.

June 3d. I cannot disentangle now the events of the last few days, nor have I a very exact idea of the numbers we have taken care of. We put two hundred and fifty on *Webster* No. 1 on Monday, among them General Devens and Colonel Briggs of Massachusetts, and, fearing that all intermediate hospitals would be full, and the weather continuing very hot, sent her, in the absence of orders, to Boston. The same day the *Vanderbilt* and *Knickerbocker* were filled, and to-day the *Spaulding*. Between two and three thousand wounded have been sent here this week, and at least nine tenths of them have been fed and cared for, as long as they remained, exclusively by the Commission.

(M.) Generally the government hospital boats are ready and glad to accept our assistance, but now and then one will stand off in the stream "all ready," needing no help, till finally, and when the sick are coming on board, at the last moment, not a pound of bread or ounce of meat will be found ready for them. The men are expected to bring rations for a day or so, in their haversacks, haversacks meanwhile being lost at the front, and men being too badly hurt to think of any such provision. . . . . . This is where the Commission comes in, and kettles of soup and tea, with fresh soft bread, gruel, and stimulants, are sent to all these boats from the tent kitchen, and with them go cups and spoons, and attendants to distribute the food. Many hundreds of men have been helped in this way, who, without such a provision, would, to say the least, have greatly suffered. Two days ago there was a hospital transport near us, "all ready," according to their own account, and after the wounded men came on board, before the first surgical case could be attended to, they had to rush over to our boat for lint, bandages, rags, pins, towels, and stimulants. One man had been without the slightest nourishment all day until an hour before his shoulder was taken off; then, when it was too late, the surgeon hurried over to ask us to take him beef-tea and egg-nog, and we crossed the coal-barges and administered it; all this after the Doctor had himself told me that morning that they needed no help. It is just the same with lint and bandages, sponges and splints, all which the Commission supplies freely. There was another boat near us with a good staff and plenty of assistants, and everything looking so fair that we supposed it all right, particularly as we were assured that she had been "preparing" for some weeks, and had "all that was necessary." All day last Sunday they were putting men on board, selecting four hundred from the five hundred sick and wounded who came down on Friday to the post hospital, and who were all received on arrival and taken care of by Dr. Ware and his assistants. When they had been put on board, and wanted food at the moment, it was not ready,—plenty of it in the rough, but nothing cooked in anticipation; and at six o'clock in the evening, as we were crossing the boat from the *Small*, which lay outside, we found the boat full of very sick men, feverish and thirsty, and calling for water, and no help at hand. We asked for basins; there were none on board; and to add to the rest, the forty "Sisters," who had come down unexpectedly, by someone's order, had all struck for keys to their staterooms, and sat about on their large trunks, forbidden to stir by the Padre, who was in a high state of ecclesiastical disgust on the deck of the *Knickerbocker*, at not finding provision made for them, including a chapel. —— labored with the indignant old gentleman upon the unreasonableness of expecting to find confessionals, &c. erected on the battle-field, but to no purpose. There sat the forty "Sisters," clean and peaceful, with their forty umbrellas and their forty baskets, fastened to their places by the Padre's eyes, and not one of them was allowed to come over and help us. So our boat's company went to work, Dr. Ware getting for us all we needed from the Commission's supplies, and before the boat left, the sickest men were washed and fed; large pails of beef-tea, milk-punch, and arrow-root were made, enough to last for the worst cases until they reached Fortress Monroe, and at half past seven we climbed over the guards to the deck of the *Small*, and the boat cast off. We wrote all the names and home addresses of the sickest men, who might be speechless on their arrival, and fastened the papers into their pockets. It was hard to have the "Sisters," who would have been so faithful, and who were so much needed, shut away from the sick men by the etiquette of their confessor. It is unpleasant to abuse people for inefficiency. Possibly they *have* all that is necessary on these government boats, stowed away in boxes somewhere, but at the precise moment when it is needed no one knows anything about it. Such boats either have no one at their head, or where there is one there are many, which is worse than none.

We have, up to this time, sent away on the Commission's boats, since Sunday, 1,770 patients. These, after having once been got upon beds, have been all methodically and tenderly cared for. The difficulties to be overcome in accomplishing it were enormous, and the greatest of them of a nature which it would now be ungrateful to describe. We have also distributed to government boats and hospitals an immense quantity of clothing and hospital stores.

(A.) Rustic Sidneys are so common we have ceased to think of it. "I guess that next fellow wants it more'n I do,"—"Won't you jus' go to that man over there first, if you please, marm; I hearn him kind o' groan jus' now; must be pretty bad hurt, I guess: I ha'n't got anythin' only a flesh-wound!" You may always hear such phrases as these repeated by one after another, as the ladies are moving on their first rounds.

There is not the slightest appearance of a conscious purpose to play the hero or the Spartan. Groans, and even yells and shrieks, are not always restrained, but complaint is never uttered, though the Irish, especially when not very severely wounded, are sometimes pathetically despondent and lachrymose, and the Frenchmen look unutterable things. But gratitude and a spirit of patience never fails, a cheerful disposition seldom. . . . . . In this republic of suffering, individuals do not often become very strongly marked in one's mind, but now and then one does so unaccountably. I am haunted by the laughing eye of a brave New Hampshire man,—laughing I am sure in agony,—whom I saw on the ——. [This was one of the worst of the government transports, badly managed, hastily loaded, and densely crowded.] He was lying closely packed among some badly wounded rebels, and in giving them some little attention I had passed him by, because he looked as if he wanted nothing, —so differently from the others. Afterwards returning that way, they seemed to have all fallen asleep; but this man's strange, cheerful eye met mine as I was carefully stepping over his feet. "Do you want anything, my man?" "Well, now you are there, I don't care if you h'ist that blanket off my leg a piece; the heft on't kind o'irks my wound." "Certainly," I said; drawing it down, and knowing at once that he must be painfully wounded; "is there nothing else I can do for you? Would n't you like a cup of water?" "If you've got some cool water handy, I should be obliged to you. I've got some in my canteen they give me this morning, but it's got warm." I brought him some, as soon as I could. "That tastes good," says he. "Do you know where this boat's goin'?" "She goes first to Fortress Monroe; whether they will send her on from there to New York, or take you ashore there, I don't know. It will be decided when you get there." "They must n't keep me there. I must go home." "Where is your home?" "It's a place called Keene, up in New Hampshire." "What's the matter with you?" "Got a ball through my thigh." "Did it touch the bone?" "Yes, broke it snap off." "Rather high up the thigh, isn't it?" "Just about as high as it can be; the doctors, they tell me,—well, first they told me tha't would kill me if they did n't take it off, and then they told me 't would kill me if they did take it off, it's so high up, they say they can't do it. So, accordin' to their account, I've got to go anyhow. That's what the doctors make out; but I'll tell you what I think: I think God Almighty's got something to say about that. If he says so, well and good, I ha'n't got nothin' to say. But I'd like to get back to Keene. They must send me. I know I'll die if they don't. They must." "I'm afraid it would hardly do to send you out to sea,—the motion of the vessel—" "O, I a'n't a bit afraid of that, I don't mind the hurt on 't. The old doctor, he was n't a goin' to send me; he said 't wan't no use, and there was n't no room. But after they'd got about loaded up, the young doctor came along, and I got hold o' him, and I told him they must send me, and finally he told 'em they must get me in somehow. That did hurt, that 'are. Fact is, I fainted away when they put me in, it hurt so. I never felt anything like that. But I tell you, when I come to and found I was rattlin' along down here, I did n't mind how much it hurt." "Is it painful now?" "Well, when they step round here, and when the engine goes, it's kinder like a jumping toothache, down there. Well, yes, it does hurt pretty bad, but I don't mind, if they'll only let me go home. I guess if they'll let me go home, I can pull through it somehow; and if I don't,—that's God Almighty's business, too; I a'n't consarned about that." And he smiled again, that brave, man to man, knowing New England smile. I found that his wound had not been dressed in three days; fortunately there was time for me to get Ware to dress it before the boat left.

(N.). . . . . We lie here just outside some other vessels at the railroad wharf. The one nearest the wharf is the *Knickerbocker* (one of our own boats, a refreshing sight to sick and well). On it we are placing the wounded as they now come in, somewhat slowly.* Since last night at ten o'clock there have been one hundred and sixty-five brought on board. This nearly completes the list of the wounded by the Saturday and Sunday engagements, excepting some two or three

*This refers to the second loading of the *Knickerbocker* after the battle.

hundred who are in a hospital on the extreme right, some ten miles from the railroad. There have now been brought in to the hospital boats about three thousand seven hundred men, of whom six or eight hundred were rebels. It has been touching to hear the expressions of surprise and gratitude from some of these young fresh-looking Southerners, as they received tender care from the hands of those who were ministering to them in their sad suffering. Of course our own wounded were carried off the field first, and this left the others with wounds for some time not dressed.

(M.) Among the sick and wounded who came on board last night were several Secessionists. One whom I was attending took my hand, with tears in his eyes: "God bless you, Miss." Another, who was near death,—he had the most terrible wound I ever saw,—said, gently: "God forgive me, honey, if it was wrong. I thought it was right, but I don't like it, that's the truth. I would rather have died for the old flag, but—I thought it was right. There, let them bury that with me" (showing me a bracelet of hair on his arm). "It's my wife's, honey; it is. My watch you may keep, and if ever the time should come when you can send it to her, please do so."

(A.) Naturally enough, the prisoners do not "bear up" as well as our own men. There is not only more whimpering, but more fretfulness and bitterness of spirit, evinced chiefly in want of regard one for another.

(N.) On board the *Commission's boats* we see the *unavoidable* miseries of war, and none other. So soon as the men come on board, all suffering except that of illness ceases, and we know and see that every comfort and every chance for recovery is freely supplied. I have a long history to tell, one of these days, of the gratefulness of the men. . . . . . I often wish,—as I give a comfort to some poor fellow, and see the sense of rest it gives him, and hear the favorite speech, "O, that's good! it's just as if mother was here,"—that the man or woman who supplied the means for the comfort were present to see how blessed it is. Believe me, you may all give and work in the earnest hope that you alleviate suffering, but none of you realize what you do,—perhaps you can't even conceive of it unless you could see your gifts *in use.* I often think of the money and supplies which, by the goodness of others, passed through my hands before I left home. How little I then knew their value! How little I then imagined that each article was to be a life-giving comfort to some one sufferer!

The object of the Commission is not clearly understood. Those who admire its noble, wise work naturally feel the wish that larger power should be given to it. But the object of the Commission itself is not this. It seeks to bring the government to do what the government *should* do for its sick and wounded. Until that object is accomplished, the Commission stands ready to throw itself into the breach, as it did during that dreadful battle-week, and as it does, more or less, all the time. The thing it asks for is not the gift of power, but that the government should come forward and take the work away from it. . . . . . There are rumors that this much-desired change will be effected. I am not afraid to say that no enterprise ever deserved better of the country than this undertaken by the Sanitary Commission. Alive to the true state of things, ever aiming at the *best* thing to be done, and striving to bring everything to bear upon that, it has already fulfilled a great work,—let those who have reaped its benefits say how great and how indispensable.

Since yesterday morning we have been leading a life which Mr. —— feels to be one of such utter discomfort that we all try to make the best of it for his sake, though I will admit to *you* that it *is* very wearing to have no proper place to eat, sit, or sleep. No matter! our *Wilson Small* will be back soon, and we shall resume our happy *home* life on the top of the old stove. We had luxury which did not please us on board the——, and piggishness which pleased us still less on board the ——, and yet we are the most cheerful set of people to be found anywhere. This morning, just as Mr.——was sitting with his head on his hand, sighing over the horrid breakfast to which we ladies had been subjected, some one looked up and spied the *Daniel Webster* coming up. Such vitality as seized us! The good *Webster*! always perfect, prompt, and true. In a moment, Dr. Grymes and Captain Bletham were on board, and did n't we shake hands all round! I suppose you know the *Webster* had to put into New York in consequence of a storm, which would have perilled the lives of many of the sick if they had pursued the voyage to Boston.

I often feel the pleasantness of our (the ladies') footing amongst all these people, official, military, naval, and medical. They clearly respect our work, and rightly appreciate it; they strengthen our hands when they can, they make no foolish speeches, but are direct and sensible in their acts and words, and when work is over, they do not feel toward us as "women with a mission," but as ladies, to be with whom is a grateful relaxation. I must say our position here is particularly proper and pleasant. . . . . . I suppose from eight to ten thousand troops have arrived here within a week. At first, I scarcely noticed their coming. I heard their gay bands, and the loud cheering of the men as the transports rounded the last bend in the river, and came in sight of the landing, but such sounds of the dreadful *other* side of war filled my ears, that, if I heard, I heeded not. For the last night or two, the arrivals by moonlight, with the cheers and the gay music, have been really enlivening. *We* see the dark side of all. You must not, however, gather only gloomy ideas from me. I see the worst—short of the actual battle-field—that can be seen. You must not allow yourself to think there is no brightness because I do not speak of it.

(M.) We have on two of our boats nine contraband women, from the Lee estate,—real Virginia "darkies," and excellent workers,—who all "wish on their souls and bodies" that the Rebels could be "put in a house together and burned up." "Mary Susan," the blackest of them, yielded at once to the allurements of freedom and fashion, and begged Mr. K.

to take a little commission for her the next time he went to Washington. "I wants you for to get me, sar, if you please, a lawn dress and hoop-skirt, sar." The women not working on our boats do the hospital washing for us in their cabins on the Lee estate, and I have been up to-day to hurry them with the *Knickerbocker's* eleven hundred pieces. The negro quarters are decent and comfortable little houses, with a wide road between them and the bank which slopes to the river. Any number of little darkey babies are rushing about, and tipping into the wash-tubs, and in one cottage we found two absurdly small babies taken care of by an antique bronze, calling itself grandmother. Babies had the measles, which would n't "come out" on one of them. So she had laid him tenderly in the open clay oven, and with hot sage-tea and an unusually large brick put to his morsels of feet, was proceeding to develop the disease. Two of the colored women and their husbands work for us at the tent kitchen, close by the shore, and entertain us by their singing. The other night Molly and Nellie collected all their friends behind their tent and commenced, in a sort of monotonous recitativo, a condensed narrative of the creation of the world; one giving out a line and all the others joining in. They went straight through from Genesis to Revelation, following with a confession of sin and exhortation to do better,—till suddenly their deep humility seemed to strike them as uncalled for, and they rose at once into the "assurance of the saints," and each one instructed her neighbor at the top of her voice to

> "Go tell all the holy angels,
> I done, done all I ever can."

Just as they came to a pause the train arrived; midnight, as usual, and the work of feeding and caring for the sick began again. Dr. Ware was busy with his nightly work of seeing that the men were properly lifted from the platform cars and put into the Sibley tents; H. was "processing" his detail with additional blankets and quilts; and Wagner, our

Zouave, and his five men, were going the rounds with hot tea and fresh bread, while we were getting ready beef-tea and punch for the use of the sickest through the night. By two o'clock we could cross the gang-plank to the *Small* again, feeling that all the men were quiet and comfortable.

We women constantly receive noble and patriotic letters from the patents [*sic*] and friends of the soldiers who have died here among us, one of our duties being to write to the families of those we have had care of. Mrs. —— had sent her the other day, from one of the —— Regiment, a little poem in such delicate acknowledgement of kindness received that I must copy it:—

"From old St. Paul till now,
Of honorable women not a few
Have left their golden ease in love to do
The saintly work that Christlike hearts pursue.

"And such an one art thou,—God's fair apostle,
Bearing his love in war's horrific train;
Thy blessed feet follow its ghastly pain,
And misery, and death, without disdain.

"To one borne from the sullen battle's roar,
Dearer the greeting of thy gentle eyes,
When he aweary, torn, and bleeding lies,
Than all the glory that the victors prize.

"When peace shall come, and homes shall smile again,
A thousand soldier-hearts in Northern climes
Shall tell their little children, with their rhymes,
Of the sweet saint who blessed the old war-times."

Chapter VI.

(A.) We were "stampeded" last night. A train arrived, and the ladies were at the kitchen ashore getting tea ready. Dr. Ware went to the cars, as usual, and two or three wounded men were brought down on litters, to be put on the *Elm City*. The doctor coming along with them said, "These men were shot on the train, just before arriving here." After they had been taken on board, M. said to me, "Do you know they are getting ready to take in the gang-plank, and are firing up on the *Elm City*?" I went on board; could not see the captain; the engineer was having the fires pushed, and said the orders had come from Colonel Ingalls, commander of the post, to fire up and get away as quickly as possible. All our boats had received the same. I went out, and with difficulty got the ladies to go on board. M., who had gone up to head-quarters to see if there was no mistake, came back with the message, "Drop down below the gunboats, at once, and look out to keep clear of vessels floating down on fire." We of course obeyed orders, knowing nothing of the reasons for them, and in half an hour all our boats were anchored a mile below, with steam up. As soon as this was accomplished, I took a yawl, and pulled back to the railroad landing, where I found everything quiet, Ware and H. taking care of the sick who had been left in the tents. Walking on to the post head-quarters, I found all the camp-followers, teamsters, sutlers, railroad and barge men, organizing in companies, and arms and ammunition serving to them. M., who had volunteered for this duty, had a company. I found the Provost-Marshal, who told me that the enemy had suddenly appeared, apparently in considerable force, about three miles from here, simultaneously on the river and the railroad. A wagon train had been captured, two or three schooners burned, the telegraph cut. It was presumed that it was an expedition designed to play havoc with this post, where there is an immense amount of army supplies of all kinds, with a force absurdly inadequate to its protection,—in fact, but a weak regiment of infantry, and a weaker one of horse; but some artillery was landing, and before day-light they would have two capital batteries of Napoleons ready, and were gathering supports. I got permission to send for the *Small*, which is short enough to be quickly handled at the landing, and to put on her the sickest of the men who had been brought down during the day to be sent to the post hospital, and who were still in tents near the landing, as it seemed to me they would suffer less disturbance afloat than ashore in case the attack was made. It was daybreak before I got them at anchor below again. At sunrise I was allowed to bring all the boats up; but as there was a standing order against the shipment of sick at this time, (in order to reserve the transports for the wounded,) we kept our patients on the *Small* for some days, the post surgeon not being able to receive them. The women were greatly annoyed and indignant at being sent, with the boats, out of harm's way.

(N.) We sat on deck. . . . . watching the fleet of transports, hospital-ships, and supply-boats hurrying after and past us, and the signaling from gunboat to gunboat, which seemed done by a lantern at the end of a long pole, dashed up and down through the darkness. It was midnight when a messenger came in the yawl, with orders to bring the *Small* back to the railroad. All the way up we worked, getting ready for as many sick as could be taken on her. Forty-five beds filled every corner of the boat, and beef-tea, punch, and gruel were ready by the time we reached the railroad-bridge. Dr. Ware and H., who had not run away, had selected the sickest of the men in the tents, and had them all ready to put on board, and with the help of the *Spaulding's* nurses, whom we called for on the way up, we took them on board that night, and the next day and the next we had them in our little boat,—some of the sickest men I ever saw,—crazy and noisy, soaked, body and mind, with swamp-poison, and in a sort of delirious remembrance of the days before the fever came,—days of mortal chill and hunger,—screaming for food, for something "hot," for "Lucifer matches" even. Two of these men died on board, not able to give their names.

The fright about the raid having somewhat subsided, we settled down again, as we supposed, into our daily routine of fitting up transports, and of receiving and feeding the sick who arrive on the trains. All sorts of messages and people are constantly coming to our tent;—surgeons from the front, to have requisitions filled for lemons and onions,* beef-stock, and brandy; orderlies, for officers sick, and just arrived to take the mail-boat, needing refreshment; and miscellaneous crowds, who have constantly to be instructed that we are not free sutlers. Captain —— had kindly provided a wall tent for our use, and Dr. Ware, in thought for our comfort, has it pitched close by our kitchen, and the sickest men arriving by train are put into it, and we are able to care for them without hurrying across the railroad track with our hot gruel. Here I found myself the other day, spoon-feeding, with a napkin under his chin, the pleasant chaplain who came down on the *Daniel Webster* to join his regiment on the first day we started as a hospital company. His turn had arrived, poor fellow, and he came back to us with a blister on each temple, and symptoms of typhoid. We had in the tent at the same time five or

*As scorbutic symptoms had been reported in certain regiments, the Commission was sending small quantities of fruit and vegetables by every returning hospital transport. It afterwards sent whole cargoes, as will be seen by reference to Appendix D.

six officers, all sick. Our little comforts, fans, slippers, mosquito-netting, napkins, cologne, are great comforts to the sick men, though to be sure one man did say to me to-day, when I put a few drops from my bottle, "*Gegenüber dem Julichs Platz*," on his handkerchief, "O my! how bad that smells! I don't mind it much, but perhaps you have spilt some of that medicine you have in your bottle!" My cologne of cologne!

The *St. Mark* arrived about this time, a splendid clipper East-Indiaman, and, after her, the *Euterpe*, both first-class new sailing vessels, entirely reconstructed interiorly by the Commission, as model hospital-ships, and having their own corps of surgeons, dressers, &c. Drawing too much water to come up the Pamunkey, they anchored at Yorktown, and the sick were taken down on steamboats to them, and they made the voyage round to New York in tow of steamers.

(A.) *June 27th*, 1862. I was intending to go down to the *St. Mark* last night. We had had some rumors the day before that Stonewall Jackson was making a dash to get in our rear, and take this post. I did not mind them, but about three o'clock, P.M., yesterday, Captain S., the active executive here, came to me, and said, privately: "Get away from this as soon as you can; the enemy is here again; our pickets are driven in, and I think we shall be obliged, within three hours, to burn everything that can't be run down the river. Give what help you conveniently can to the vessels on the river as you go down, but don't stop this side of Cumberland." I called in our men and women, found that our machinery, which had been repairing for two days, was in such disorder that it could only be used at all by the exertions of three men supplying the place of certain fractured iron, with their arms; and then but very slowly, and with great care, of course. We were in no condition to help anybody else. I pushed off, however, in quarter of an hour, taking the *Wissahickon* and *Elizabeth* in company. One or two boats started before us, and several immediately after. As we passed down, we found the gunboats with their boardingnettings up, and all ready for action, and the skirt of wood along the shore of the White House grounds cut away to allow a sweep to their guns. We left our consorts at Cumberland to take forage vessels in tow down, and went on slowly to West Point, where we anchored. Soon after noon to-day the Captain reported his machinery repaired, and we started to return to White House. The river was full of vessels coming down. We could learn nothing from them except that everything had been ordered to "clear out." We got here about sunset, and found almost everything gone,—a remarkably orderly and successful removal of a vast amount of stores. Among what remained, whiskey and hay were distributed, and everything was ready for firing.

Stonewall Jackson had not come down upon us as we had supposed, but our right wing had been turned, and the enemy was hourly expected to be pushing into White House. The authorities at "Head-quarters" were by no means as much surprised as we were at it all. Every preparation had been quietly making for several days for the arrival of the enemy, and the evacuation and repossession were effected in as neat and complete a manner as if the affair had been arranged between the parties by the penny-post.

The *Knickerbocker*, and other of our boats, just as they were, were used as retreats for railroad men and straggling Northerners, exclusive of sutlers. The government boats, with the *Commodore, Daniel Webster*, &c., were ordered up, and the fifteen hundred sick men from the shore hospital put on board. The Sisters of Charity, who had been for a few days occupying the White House, were distributed through the different government craft, glad now to do what they could; and so, all in good order, the hospital ships, one after another, departed, the *Wilson Small* lingering as long as possible, till the telegraph wires had been cut, and the enemy announced by mounted messenger to be at "Tunstall's," worried constantly in his advance by Stoneman with his cavalry, till all should have got safely off, when he would fall back towards Williamsburg, and the rebels would walk into our deserted places.

So we came away,—watching the moving off of the last transports and barges, and of the *Canonicus*, head-quarters' boat, with Colonel Ingalls and Captain Sawtelle and General Casey and staff. . . . . . But by far the most interesting incident was the spontaneous movement of the slaves, who, when it was known that the Yankees were running away, came flocking from all the country about, bringing their little movables, frying-pans and old hats and bundles, to the riverside. There was no more appearance of anxiety or excitement among them than among the soldiers themselves. Fortunately there was plenty of deck-room for them on the forage boats, one of which, as we passed it, seemed filled with women only, in their gayest dresses and brightest turbans, like a whole load of tulips for a horticultural show. The black smoke began to rise from the burning stores left on shore, and now and then the roar of the battle came to us, but they were quietly nursing their children and singing hymns. The day of their deliverance had come, and they accepted this most wonderful change in absolute placidity.

All night we sat on the deck of the *Small*, slowly moving away, watching the constantly increasing cloud, and the fire-flashes over the trees toward White House; watching the fading out of what had been to us, through these strange weeks, a sort of home where we had all worked together and been happy,—a place which is sacred to some of us now, from its intense, living remembrances, and for the hallowing of them all by the memory of one who through months of death and darkness lived and worked in self-abnegation,—lived in, and for, the sufferings of others, and finally gave himself a sacrifice for them.

Appendix

Appendix A.

See page 55.

"The Commission is at this time actually distributing daily, of hospital supplies, much more than the government."

This refers to a temporary emergency alone, for, notwithstanding the recognized necessity for volunteer aid, it is believed that the aggregate of all hospital supplies voluntarily furnished by the people through the Sanitary Commission and otherwise, great and unparalleled as this gratuitous supply is, is but about one tenth as much as is furnished by government. This fact ought to be kept in mind, as there is a natural tendency on the part of those who are rendering volunteer aid to exaggerate the relative magnitude of their own labors, while the permanent and vastly larger provisions of government are underrated, and a habit of unjust censure indulged in, in speaking of deficiencies which have to be supplied. The character of this censure generally indicates complete ignorance of the failures of other governments when engaged in war, and a careless estimate of the immense labors involved, and difficulties which invariably have to be overcome, in providing for the constant necessities and exigencies of a great army. It is the opinion of those whose sympathies with the suffering of the soldiers on the one hand, and whose careful study of facts on the other, ought to give weight to their judgments, that never before, in the world's history, was an army so well cared for in all its departments, Quartermaster's, Commissary, and Medical, and that never before, when deficiencies were discovered, were they, on an average, as speedily remedied. In every great trial, by war, of a nation, it has been found necessary to employ a very large number of men in positions of the gravest responsibility, for which they were not adapted by nature or by training. This involves, of course, not only incompetency for duties assumed, but necessarily opens a door to continued neglect of trusts, frauds, and peculations, which, under ordinary circumstances, would seem to be of stupendous magnitude. This is always a part of the cost of war, and, so far from being the peculiarity of a republican form of government, or of the present occasion, in no modern war have frauds and inefficiency of administrative service been anything like as slightly manifested in the condition and efficiency, under all circumstances, of the troops in the field; and this, whether we have regard to their food, clothing, equipments, transportation, or, finally, to the provision which has existed for the sick and wounded. The sustained average health, vigor, and good spirits of our several grand armies, in the great variety of circumstances in which they have been placed, tells of a virtue and a vital force in our people and in our institutions, which, rightly understood, should put to shame much customary cavilling of flippant critics.

The writer of this note has recently travelled through a region larger than the whole of England, which a year before his visit was held by one hundred and fifty thousand rebels in arms, and with advantages for defensive warfare such as no country of equal extent in Europe possesses. In every mile of this road he saw traces of the desperate fanaticism of personal ambition and pride, reckless of the life and property of others, with which its defense had been conducted. And beyond it he found those who were re-establishing the supremacy of republican law in this land. He spent more than a week with them, and in that time he heard no complaint so frequent or so bitter as that against the whimperers and mischief-makers they had left behind. The health and patience of the men was a matter of profound astonishment to him. That the officers were many of them exceedingly unfit for their responsibility cannot be denied. In what army are not many of the officers found to be so? But even this was chiefly to be attributed to the very influence which, in its worst form, was made the cloak of the conspiracy which brought about the rebellion, and was commonly felt and said to be so. And thus the army, fighting the open, fights also with the insidious enemies of the country, and when it returns both will have been conquered. But if incompentency is common among State-appointed officers, what evidence does the condition of the army give of the action of great talent, integrity, industry, and patriotic zeal, in the manner in which it is provided for! Nowhere did the writer fail to find the men clothed and fed as never were soldiers clothed and fed in the pettiest frontier war before. He reached a division in the extreme advance; bivouacked in a swamp, its wounded picket-guardsmen were being brought in and cared for, methodically, and well; not with the refinement of a civilized home, but as wounded soldiers seldom have been in the history of wars, under the most favorable circumstances, before in the world. There was nothing which, thus situated, the surgeon could wish to have with him, which he had not. This division, since it came to the war, had marched over four thousand miles, and fought six great battles, and now here in the swamp, wading from hammock to hammock, the enemy in force in the next really dry land, the men looked as well in health, and as cheerful in spirits, as a company of harvesters at their mooning. They were carefully examined. Were they in want of clothing? No. Were they well shod? Yes. Were they well fed? They had full rations, and could ask for nothing better. What did they want? "To finish up the business they came here for, and go home." Nothing else. It was actually so there at the advanced post in the swamp, and it was so—it is so at this moment—

wherever, on sea or ashore, the seven hundred thousand men now employed by our government are scattered at their work. By what despotic power was a machine ever made that could have accomplished this, in two years?

F. L. O.

Appendix B.

See page 67.

REGULATIONS FOR FLOATING HOSPITAL SERVICE OF THE SANITARY COMMISSION, FOR THE CAMPAIGN IN VIRGINIA.

TERMS OF SERVICE.

The Sanitary Commission, being itself under military authority, in order to meet its responsibilities, must require of all persons who engage in the hospital service of the army under its direction, that they place themselves, for the time being, entirely at its disposal.

Those who volunteer their services gratuitously being supposed to do so fully and in good faith, no distinction can be known between them and those who may be paid for their services, it being understood that these services, in both cases, once engaged or accepted, are to be claimed equally of right by the Commission.

ADMINISTRATION.

An agent of administration for the Commission will be appointed for each hospital vessel, who will be regarded by those on board as responsible for her fittings and supplies.

WARDS.

Each vessel will be divided into hospital wards, designed each for the accommodation of from fifty to one hundred and fifty patients. In case of convalescents, a larger number will be properly included in a ward.

SURGEONS.

A surgeon in charge will be appointed to each vessel, who will be responsible for the reception, classification, and distribution of patients in the wards. He will sign any necessary official medical reports of the vessel. Each ward will be placed under the especial charge of one surgeon, and, if practicable, there will be a surgeon for each ward.

ASSISTANTS TO SURGEONS.

An assistant to the surgeon (with the title of Ward-master) is to be constantly on duty in each ward. Under instructions from the surgeon of the ward, he will superintend and be responsible for the entire treatment of the patients of the ward, during the hours in which he is appointed to be on duty.

NURSES.

Two or more nurses are to be constantly on duty in each ward. They will perform any and all duties necessary in the care of the patients, under instructions from the surgeons received through the ward-masters.

DISPENSARY.

A dispensary will be established on each vessel, and one or more apothecaries will be placed in charge of it. They will be responsible for the medical stores, and for their proper compounding and issue upon requisitions of the surgeons through the ward-masters.

HOSPITAL PANTRY AND LINEN CLOSET.

These will be in charge of ladies, who will issue to ward-masters or nurses, or themselves administer and dispense, under proper control of the surgeons, special diet and drink, and articles of bed and personal clothing for the patients.

WATCHES.

Ward-masters and nurses, and all who have part in duty of a constant character, will be divided into two watches, which will be on duty alternately, as follows:—

1.	From 7 A.M.	to	1 P.M.	A
2.	" 1 P.M.	to	4 P.M.	B (dog watch.)
3.	" 4 P.M.	to	7 P.M.	A " "
4.	" 7 P.M.	to	1 A.M.	B
5.	" 1 A.M.	to	7 A.M.	A
6.	" 7 A.M.	to	1 P.M.	B (second day.)

TIMES OF MEALS.

BREAKFAST.

One watch at 6.40 A.M. (being then off duty.)
The other at 7 A.M. " "

DINNER.

One watch at 12.30 P.M. " "
The other at 1.15 P.M. " "

TEA.

One watch at 6.40 P.M. " "
The other at 7.00 P.M. " "

HOUSE DIET.

BREAKFAST.

To be ready at 7 A.M.
Bread (or Toast) with Butter.
Coffee or Tea.

10

DINNER.

To be ready at 1.15 P.M.
Beef Soup and Boiled Beef or Beef Stew.
Boiled Rice or Hominy.
Bread or Crackers.

TEA.

To be ready at 7 P.M.
Bread or Toast or Crackers, with Butter.
Coffee or Tea.

When practicable, the house diet will be served at tables to such patients as are able to come to them. When not practicable to arrange tables, such patients as may be designated by the surgeons will be divided into squads of forty, and a squad-master appointed to each, who will receive and distribute to the rest the prepared diet, as may be found most convenient. Patients not able to leave their beds will not be included in these squads, but house diet will be served to them by the nurses of their wards, if ordered by the surgeon.

SPECIAL DIET.

The surgeons will ascertain from the administrative agent, or from the ladies, what articles of diet are available on the vessel, and in their morning rounds direct what choice shall be made from these for the diet of each patient, for whom the house diet would not be suitable, during the succeeding twenty-four hours. The ward-master on duty at the hour for surgeons' morning rounds will, in regular order, be on duty at each meal-time during the following twenty-four hours, and will consequently be able to direct the entire diet of each patient from verbal instructions. He should, as soon as possible, notify the proper person (no rule in this respect being practicable for all vessels) of the quantity of each article of special diet which will be required at each meal in his ward, and the proper time should (if necessary) send the nurses it, and see it properly distributed.

SURGEONS' ROUNDS.

Surgeons' rounds should commence at 9 A.M., and at 6 P.M. The ward-master on duty will closely attend the surgeon, and receive his instructions as he passes through his ward. The ward-master off duty may also attend the surgeon at this time, for the benefit of receiving instructions directly. The surgeon may make this his duty, otherwise it will be optional.

ALL HANDS.

In receiving and discharging patients, or in any emergency which makes it necessary, ward-masters and nurses may be required to do duty in their watches off. In cleaning, fitting, or repairing the vessel for hospital purposes, they will act under orders of the administrative agent.

RECEIVING AND DISTRIBUTING PATIENTS.

Before patients are taken on board, the vessel should be properly moored or placed, gangways or other means of entrance arranged, and, if possible, all duties completed, for the time being, in the performance of which the crew of the vessel are required. The surgeon, who should have previously informed himself of the character of the accommodations for patients in all parts of each ward, should detail a sufficient number of guides and bearers to convey the patients, and of all necessary attendants at the gangway, and within the wards. These should remove their boots, and each squad of bearers should be instructed that all orders will be given them by their guide alone, and that no one else is to speak aloud while carrying a patient, or passing through the wards. All persons not having a specified duty to perform in receiving patients, should be put where they will not be in the way or disturb the patients, but where they can be readily called on if the force engaged is found insufficient.

As each patient is brought on board, he will be examined by the surgeon in charge, who will direct where he shall be taken; at the same time notes will be taken, as follows:—*Number, Name, Company, Regiment, Residence, Remarks.*

The administrative agent will, at the same time, cause a corresponding number to be placed on the effects of the patient, which he will take care of, to be returned to the patient on his leaving the vessel. If practicable, the patients may, before being taken to their berths or cots, be washed and supplied with clean clothing.

It will not usually be in the power of the surgeon in charge to select patients for his vessel. It may, however, be proper for him to protest against taking patients whose illness is not of a sufficiently serious character to warrant their withdrawal from the seat of war, or those for whose cases there is less suitable provision on the vessel than in the hospitals they are leaving, or those already in a dying condition, whose end will have been accelerated or whose suffering aggravated by their removal; also, when going to sea, against taking cases of compound fracture of the lower extremities.

FRED. LAW OLMSTED, *Gen'l Sec'y.*

White House, Virginia, May 20, 1862.

SANITARY COMMISSION.
Atlantic Hospital Transport Service.

THE REGULATION OF DIET FOR PATIENTS.

The simplest possible arrangements should be made for the diet of patients which will be consistent with their proper treatment.

At the outset, the cook may be ordered to prepare daily for breakfast, to be ready at 7 A.M., ten gallons of tea and fifteen loaves of bread in slices, with butter, for every hundred patients on board; for dinner, ten gallons of beef-stew made with vegetables, and fifteen loaves of bread, for every hundred patients on board; for tea, the same as for breakfast.

Orders for special diet should, as far as possible, be confined to beef-tea, arrow-root or farina gruel, milk-porridge, and milk-punch.

Quantities of each of these articles, except the punch, may be prepared by the cook once a day, and delivered to the matron, under whose care they should be warmed in portions over spirit-lamps, as required at any time during the day or night.

As a general rule, for each hundred patients on board, there should be prepared, for twenty-four hours,—

2 1/2 gallons of beef-tea,
4 gallons of gruel,
1/2 gallon of milk-porridge.

Where the patients are chiefly suffering from illness, especially if from fevers, the above quantities will be found larger than is necessary. Where a large proportion of them are severely wounded, they may need to be slightly increased.

By estimating the quantity of each article which will be required for the twenty-four hours, as thus instructed, the surgeon in charge will find it best to give his orders to the cook for everything at once, one day in advance.

If the quantities ordered prove too small, the deficiency can be made good by the matron with crackers, tea, canned meats, or meat essence, &c., in the pantry; it being best, if possible, to avoid any call upon the cook or the ship's kitchen for this purpose.

If the quantities prove too large for one day, the saving can be used the next. Whether too large or too small, a proper modification can be readily made in the order to the cook for the remainder of the trip. The surgeon in charge will in this way be relieved of the necessity of giving further consideration to this department of administration, which, if not thus simplified, will be found to be a source of much trouble and anxiety, greatly withdrawing his attention from surgical and medical duties proper. Associated surgeons should be careful to make no demands for diet, inconsistent with this arrangement.

Milk-punch is best made with cold water in the pantry. This and all other cold drinks can be made under the superintendence of the matron, without any call upon the cook. The cook should, however, be required to keep a supply, as large as convenient, of hot water, constantly ready to meet any demand from a surgeon or the matron.

Appendix C.

See page 104.

Copy of Letter to the Medical Director of the Army of the Potomac.

White House, Va., June 3, 1862.

My Dear Sir:—There must be some frightful misunderstanding at the bottom of what is occurring here, in your department. It is obvious from the tenor of your telegraphic communications to me, that you are altogether wrongly informed about it. The Sanitary Commission, let me say at once, has not only obeyed every order, no matter how irregular or disrespectful the mode of its transmission, but has in good faith endeavored to carry out, at every point it could reach, what was judged to be *your intention*, supplying the absence or neglect of other agents on whom you appeared to depend, as it best could. Till night before last it made itself subordinate to the Surgeon-General of Pennsylvania, who assumed to act as your aid, and, under positive orders given by him in your name, it refrained from pursuing a plan previously approved by you, and by following which it is now obvious that a much greater and safer transport of the wounded would have occurred. From Sunday night to the present time, the Surgeon-General of Pennsylvania has not been seen here; a thousand wounded men have, in the meantime, arrived, and, as far as I am informed, not the slightest provision of any kind has been made for them under order from you, or by any one whom you have regarded as under your orders, except the Sanitary Commission. After waiting some hours yesterday morning for the Surgeon-General of Pennsylvania (who till then had been in charge of the railroad wharf) to act, finding men fainting in the sun ashore, I assumed the responsibility of taking eighty of them upon our little boat, and of having the remainder brought on the *Daniel Webster* No. 2. After doing so, I found one Dr. ——, very hard at work dressing wounded, &c. By advice of Captain Sawtelle and myself, he took provisional medical charge, and I then telegraphed you, advising that Dr. —— or Dr. —— should be placed in general charge, with discretionary powers.

We were doing what we could with men and women who could be spared from our boats, which were all full of wounded, to provide for those on the *Webster* and ashore. Before night, the *Spaulding* having arrived, I brought up fourteen fresh men and the ladies, with two physicians, and they have been steadily at work, and up to this time (noon of Tuesday) operating, dressing, feeding, and, with the assistance of other volunteers, bringing the wounded from the cars to the boat.

The *Vanderbilt* came more than a week ago, empty, and assigned to hospital service. She came to the wharf that had been built, at my request, for the use of the Sanitary Commission, refused to leave at my request, and has occupied it to our exclusion ever since. She has had surgeons and a large detail of soldiers on board, and I had been informed that she was reserved for the transportation of wounded, by your orders. Neither those on board of her nor those at the camp hospital appeared at the railroad, or lent any assistance, to my knowledge, to the care of the wounded, until, under advice from Captain Sawtelle and myself, Dr. ——, who had received your telegram disacknowledging him as having any official position, requested the surgeon in charge to bring the

Vanderbilt to the railroad wharf. Having our boats and the removal of the wounded in ambulance trains to attend to, I did not think it necessary to inquire if she were prepared for hospital duty, knowing that she had been a week idle, and previously in hospital service; but late this morning I was informed that she had not any commissary, or even necessary medical stores on board, and nothing whatever was being prepared for the sustenance of the patients.

We have provided bread and molasses, for the want of anything else ready. We have been also called upon for, and are providing, lint and bandages, &c., &c.

The *Elm City* and *Knickerbocker* are both off, the *Spaulding* is yet to discharge the commissary stores with which she came loaded, and there is not a boat here now which can carry wounded, nor is there a tent pitched for them.

I have no time to be more full and exact. I have called on Colonel Ingalls to establish a cooking arrangement on shore, and shall try to get beef for soup.

I hear that more wounded are arriving. God knows what will be done with them.

As the telegraph refuses to send any messages to you to-day, being fully occupied with the General's business, I shall, if possible, send this to you this evening by a special messenger.

I am very faithfully, &c.

Copy of a Letter to the Surgeon-General.

Steamboat Wilson Small,
Off White House, Va., June 17, 1862.

(A.) My Dear General:—Your prompt action, of which I am notified by your telegram of this date, in securing the shipment of large supplies of anti-scorbutics to the Army of the Potomac, without waiting for the Medical Director to assume the responsibility of ordering them, leads me to hope that you may think it right in like manner to interpose for the protection of the army from other evils, for which the remedies are equally obvious, and more readily attainable.

I therefore urge that tarpaulings, old sails, felt, or canvas in bolts, with means of putting it together, be sent here immediately, in quantities sufficient to form a shelter for ten thousand wounded men. The materials for extending and supporting it in the form of sheds can be found in the woods immediately in the rear of the line of operations, where the shelters should be placed. I should propose that at least one depot for wounded should in this way be prepared for each army corps. Water should be secured in its vicinity, and means for providing large quantities of beef-tea or soup.

I know that such an arrangement would have saved many hundred lives after the battle of Fair Oaks. Nearly all of those with whom I conversed, of the first three thousand wounded men who received aid at this point from the Sanitary Commission, assured me that they had been without shelter from sun or rain, and without nourishment, from the time they fell until they came into our hands. This would be a period of from one to four days. The men seemed sincere, and their appearance was such as to lead me to the conclusion that, in many cases, at least, they asserted no more than the truth.

If, without waiting for a demand from the Medical Director, or the convenience of the Quartermaster's staff of this army, it would be in your power to order it, it seems to me that a provision of the kind I have indicated should be made within a single week. Everything necessary should be sent here; canvas, nails, tools, laborers, kettles, beef, pans, spoons, cooks. The smallest service for hospital purposes cannot be procured here now by the most energetic and persistent surgeons in less than a fortnight from the time they undertake to secure it. I have called three times a day, for ten days, for a detail of ten men to police the landing-place of the hospital boats; and though constantly promised me, and though the need for the work is acknowledged to be very great, I do not yet succeed in getting them.

Memorandum of Arrangements proposed by the Secretary of the Commission, to prevent a recurrence of the confusion in the Transport Service which occurred after the Battle of Fair Oaks.

The following is a list of Transports understood to be at present available for hospital service for the Army of the Potomac:—

Sea Steamers, fitted for long passages outside.

S. R. Spaulding.	Daniel Webster No. 1.

Coast-Steamers, which must make a harbor on the approach of bad weather, and which should not be sent beyond Philadelphia, unless the necessity is urgent.

Elm City,	Commodore,
State of Maine,	Kennebeck,
John Brooks,	Daniel Webster No. 2.

Coast-Steamers which should not be run outside.

Vanderbilt,	Louisiana,
Whilldin,	Knickerbocker.

Sailing vessels adapted to be used as Stationary Hospitals, or to be towed outside.

St. Mark.	Euterpe.

The aggregate capacity of these vessels is equal to the accommodation of four thousand (4,000) patients, and may be increased to five thousand (5,000) if the necessity is urgent.

From the time a boat leaves, until she can be prepared to leave again,—

will be, if she	runs		to New York,	7 days,
"	"	"	to Philadelphia,	6 days,
"	"	"	to Washington,	4 days,
"	"	"	to Annapolis,	4 days,
"	"	"	to Baltimore,	4 days,
"	"	"	to Old Point,	2 days.

If, in the event of a general engagement, all the wounded sent from White House are taken to the nearest hospitals, until these are full, there will be occupation for but few of the boats; four of them, for instance, would take seven hundred (700) a day to Fortress Monroe continuously. Having filled the nearer hospitals, however, all the vessels would be insufficient to sustain a continuous movement to those more distant. Moreover, most of the transports are unfit to convey patients to the most distant hospitals. It is, therefore, necessary that the business should be so arranged that transports may, from the beginning, run both to the nearer and the more distant hospitals, and that the limited number of sea-going vessels should be run only to the distant seaports.

To accomplish this, I suggest that the different transports be formed into *lines*, as follows:—

1. For *Virginia* hospitals.

(Fortress Monroe, Newport's News, Portsmouth, and Point Lookout.)

2. For *Maryland* hospitals.

(Washington, Alexandria, Annapolis, and Baltimore.)

3. For *Pennsylvania* hospitals.

4. For *New York* hospitals.

As two of the sea-going vessels cannot come up to White House, and these, to be used effectively, must be towed by the other two, the New York line would be best employed in preventing too great an accumulation at Fortress Monroe,—running only from Fortress Monroe to New York.

If it be assumed that seven hundred (700) will arrive daily at White House, they may be disposed of according to the accompanying schedule with regularity, and with no necessity for crowding.

Plan for the Disposition of Patients to be Sent in Hospital Transports from White House.

Days	Hospital	Men.	Md.	Va.	Penn.	N.Y.	
1st day	Va.	300		300			
" "	Md.	400	400				1st day, 700
2nd day	Penn.	400					
" "	Va.	300		600		600	2d " 1,400
3rd day	Md.	400	800				
" "	Va.	300		300			3d " 2,100
4th day	Md.	400	1,200				
" "	Va.	300		135			4th " 2,800
5th day	Md.	400	1,600				
" "	Va.	300		435			5th " 3,500
6th day	Md.	400	2,000				
" "	Va.	300		735		1,665	6th " 4,200
7th day	Va.	300		1,035			
" "	Penn.	400					7th " 4,800
8th day	Va.	300		735			
" "	Md.	400	2,400		800		8th " 5,600
9th day	Va.	300		1,035			
" "	Md.	400	2,800				9th " 6,300
10th day	Va.	300		1,335			
" "	Md.	400	3,200				10th " 7,000
11th day	Va.	300		1,170		2,130	
" "	Md.	400	3,600				11th " 7,700
12th day	Va.	300		1,470			
" "	Md.	400	4,000				12th " 8,400
13th day	Va.	300		1,700			
" "	Md.	400	4,400				13th " 9,100
14th day	Penn.	400			1,200		
" "	Va.	300		2,070			14th " 9,800
15th day	Md.	400	4,800				
" "	Va.	300		2,370			15th " 10,500
16th day	Md.	400	5,200			2,730	
" "	Va.	300		2,070			16th " 11,200
TOTAL		11,200	5,200	2,070	1,200	2,730	11,200

To carry out the foregoing plan, the *Kennebeck* and *Daniel Webster* No. 2 should be run exclusively to the Virginia hospitals,—one daily, each carrying three hundred (300) patients at a trip.

The *Commodore, Vanderbilt, State of Maine,* and *Louisiana* should be run exclusively to the Maryland hospitals, each carrying four hundred (400) patients at a trip, one daily, the round trip being four days.

The *Elm City*, being the best of the coast boats for outside work, would run to the nearest outside post, Philadelphia, once every six days, conveying four hundred (400) at each trip.

The *John Brooks*, the *Whilldin*, and the *Knickerbocker* would be surgical receiving hospitals, or reserve boats, to take the place of any detained by grounding or other accident.

The vessels of the New York line can be diverted to Philadelphia as often as it is thought desirable.

After the wounded have ceased coming to White House, the vessels of the New York line can be run to other more Northern and Eastern ports, until the nearer hospitals are emptied.

The above presumes that cases of light wounds and of extremely severe wounds will not be allowed to come to White House at all.

Respectfully,

(Signed,) FRED. LAW OLMSTED,
Gen'l Sec'y Sa n. Com.

Appendix D.

See page 125.

Shortly after the battle of Fair Oaks, the new and vastly more provident, liberal, and wisely economical policy introduced into the medical service, with the appointment of Dr. Hammond as Surgeon-General, and of the new corps of Medical Inspectors, began to be felt in the army of the Potomac,—and although many of the agents necessary to the perfect success of that policy were unable at once to accommodate their habits to the required change, the Commission, scrupulously adhering to its purpose to do nothing which the properly responsible officials in any department evinced any readiness to do without its assistance, had the satisfaction of seeing the necessity for its special service, in connection with the hospital transports, grow gradually smaller and smaller. Under the dry, taciturn, and impenetrable manner, promising nothing, of the new Medical Director of the Army of the Potomac, who, just after the battle of the Seven Days, relieved a predecessor of precisely the opposite qualities, was found to be concealed some influence by means of which whatever had before been impossible began to be thought possible, and to be tried for, after a few judicious dismissals had been made; and, after a few visits of influential friends to Governors and Senators in behalf of the dismissed had resulted in nothing but an incomprehensible failure of their purpose, the Commission's occupation was more than half gone with that army. But where so many agents are to be depended on, and such sudden new dispositions and reorganizations must be made, as after those terrible seven days, it is impossible that any demand of a large army should always be promptly and fully met. Anxiety for the well, that they might be saved from disease, soon outweighed anxiety lest the sick should not be tenderly cared for, and in more than one direction an opportunity was found to supply temporary deficiencies, which otherwise would have told severely upon the health of many thousand men. During the month after the army reached and intrenched itself on the James River, the vessels managed by the Commission probably did a better service in what they brought to the army, than in the comfort they secured to the sick who were sent away upon them. The following extracts will serve to give the reader a more complete understanding of its ruling spirit and purpose, and show its continued action to the time of the withdrawal of the army of the Potomac from the Peninsula.

(A.) *Norfolk, June 30, 1862.*—We were driven from White House Friday P.M.; arrived at Old Point yesterday. Being unable to get coal there, came here this evening. Shall coal to-night and leave at daybreak for Harrison's Bar, on James River, where the gunboats are said to be. We hope to get further up, but are advised by General Dix that we cannot safely attempt it at present.

(A.) *Off Berkeley, James River, July 1, 1862.*—We felt our way up the river slowly, and with some difficulty, having no pilot, and seeing no vessel under way after passing out of sight of Newport's News until we reached this point. Here there was a gunboat and three small steam-transports, each of which afterwards left, so that for a short time we were alone. Transports soon began to come up, however, and to-night there are a dozen or more about us.

We have Colonel ——, Colonel ——, and a few other wounded officers on board. They were sent to us by General McClellan's own ambulance, half an hour after we arrived. The General had been here, and left only as we were coming to the wharf. The officers he saw here converse with us freely, and we have had officers on board from most of the army corps, who have also talked, apparently without reserve, with us. Yet reports and opinions are so contradictory, that we are in singular uncertainty as to what has happened and as to what we have to expect.

The officers and soldiers all show the influence of intense excitement; they acknowledge the gravest anxiety; they are terribly fatigued, yet generally seem in good spirits. They speak much of the bravery of the men.

(A.) *Chesapeake Bay, July 4, 1862.*—I left our anchorage off Head-quarters of the Army of the Potomac, where I wrote you last, about four o'clock yesterday afternoon, and am running to Washington, by request of the Medical Director, to advise the Surgeon-General of the sanitary condition of the army, and to secure the immediate supply, as far as possible, of its most urgent surgical and medical wants. As the rebels have put out the lights, and we could get no pilot, we were all night feeling our way down the river, and shall not be able, with all we can do, to get to Washington till late to-night. I hope to get what is most necessary, and leave on our return before night to-morrow. I telegraphed from Old Point to have everything advanced.

I have seen and conversed freely with many staff officers, and been among the men, wounded and well—if any can be called well, where all are feverish with seven days and nights of fatigue and exhaustion and starvation and excitement. One, a Major-General, said, "I have not been asleep, nor have I tasted food, in five days. I have only sustained myself with coffee and cigars." As to the men, the following is a fair sample of statements commonly made: "My regiment has had, for the last five days before arriving here, two days' rations; what has been eaten of this has been uncooked; during that time it has made five hard marches, and fought five battles; one third of it has fallen in killed or wounded, and not one man has been shot in the back. One third of what remains is now on picket duty in the woods, which the enemy is shelling; the other lies yonder, in the mud, sleeping on its arms." This was during the rain, which fell in such torrents day before yesterday. Yesterday the enemy was attacking again, and the whole army in the line of battle up to the time we left.

The exultant confidence of the army in itself is beyond all verbal expression. It has grown out of the experience of its ability to resist and foil and terribly punish desperate assaults made upon it, as is supposed with forces greatly superior in number. It says, proudly, "All that men can do, we can do." But there is also the consciousness of a terrible strain upon its energies, of an unnatural strength, and the reflection is frequent that there must be a limit to every man's endurance.

Rest and recuperation,—how are they to be had? The first only by the relief of reinforcements; the second only by good diet and favorable hygienic circumstances. Eastern Virginia is all malarious,—the banks of James River notoriously so; the army is chiefly upon a moderately elevated, slightly undulating table-land; the river on the south side; swampy ground at no great distance on the other sides. It is open, airy, dry,—a healthful point, upon the whole, as any that could be selected east of Richmond. But the sun will lie exceedingly fierce upon it, and it is supposed the army has lost two thirds of its tents. Probably a majority of the men have lost also their knapsacks and blankets. Many were without caps or shoes. The area held is small, and will be crowded. If the enemy is active, as it would appear his policy to be, the officers will be too much occupied with the immediate military necessities of the position to give much attention to police duties. Even if they should be well disposed, the excessively fatigued and exhausted condition of the men, and the necessity of reserving their strength from day to day for the struggle with the enemy, will forbid the constant labor which would be necessary to prevent a terrible accumulation of nuisances, until at least reinforcements shall arrive so large that no more than the ordinary quotas will be required for guard and picket duty. After such tension and trial, a rapid reduction of force must also occur from sickness, and those not on the sick-list will suffer from the lassitude of reaction from excitement. Under these circumstances, all our experience shows that it will be hardly possible to enforce requirements, the observance of which must be essential to a healthy camp.

Unless large reinforcements speedily arrive, then, not only must the army feel that its heroism is unappreciated, and the object for which it struggled is to be lost by the neglect of others, and thus become dejected, dispirited, and morally resistless to the dangers of disease; but it will be physically impossible to establish such guards against these dangers as are most obviously and directly called for.

There is, in general, a large degree of confidence that, with the aid of the gunboats, which are throwing shell on the flanks at frequent intervals, we can hold the position till sufficient reinforcements come to place it beyond question; but no one speaks with entire confidence, and the nearer to the head the graver seems the apprehension,—though with all there is that strange exultation—ready to break out in laughter, like a crazy man's. There are some few who are utterly despondent and fault-finding. But there is less of this than ever before, and fewer stragglers and obvious cowards, nothing like what was seen after Pittsburg Landing. Of what we saw after Bull Run there is not the slightest symptom. In short, we have then a real grand army, tried, enduring, heroic,—worth all we can give to save it.

(C.) On Saturday we commenced the distribution of the cargo, and it has been going steadily on since in a very gratifying manner, every one concerned throwing off his coat, and working with a will, these intensely hot days,—surgeons, quartermasters, and other officers, always giving us every possible assistance in their eagerness to get this agreeable addition to their fare into the camp-kettles as soon as possible. The salted fish was a grand hit. It seems to have a peculiar attraction for languid appetites in this hot weather. We have met, thus far, with but one man inclined to throw any obstruction in the way of the distribution,—a brigade commissary, who seemed to think any unusual indulgence of a soldier's whims of appetite must be demoralizing. Word of our intention had gone through the brigade, however, before he interfered, and the eagerness of the surgeons and of the soldiers took him very quickly out of the way without any efforts on our part. Regimental transportation was quickly at the wharf, with the thanks and compliments of the colonels, and each received its quota. . . . . . The promptness with which the cargo—nearly a thousand barrels—would have been discharged, will be somewhat affected by the inability of some of the regiments of Heintzelman's corps to send transportation, on account of a movement for which they are ordered to stand in readiness to-day. . . . . . The sudden orders given yesterday for the immediate transportation of several thousand sick, have caused an influx of sick to the landing, overrunning all that the exertions of the Medical Director could do to provide for them. . . . . . This morning we found five hundred and sixty convalescents on board the transport *Cahawba*, with, to use the language of the ——, "not a bit of a thing aboard for 'em to chaw upon." As the poor fellows, many of them just getting up from fever, had been, in most cases, finding their way from the camps to the landing on foot, during the night, their want was urgent. Fortunately, we had a good supply of the concentrated beef of Martinez's preparation, and were not long in getting ready an excellent breakfast for them. It is in just such cases as this, where misery is massed, and where what is done tells not only for the relief of misery, but for the strength of the army and the putting down of the rebellion, that we find the greatest satisfaction in stepping in with the gifts of the people. Many of these men were in just the condition in which a set-back would be likely to lead to a relapse and lingering illness, and in which again, if they were well cared for, they might be built up rapidly, and soon be sent back to their muskets.

On account of the movements to-day, I shall ride out to the camps this afternoon, and make some change of arrangements for the further distribution of the anti-scorbutics. The gunboats were playing very lively at sunrise, a little way down the river. This is as much as I should say to-day, but you will hear of something that you hardly expect by the next mail-boat.

Cambridge: Stereotyped and Printed by Welch, Bigelow, & Co.

Index